COMPACT *Research*

Acne and Skin Disorders

Peggy J. Parks

Diseases and Disorders

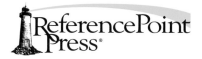

ReferencePoint Press®

San Diego, CA

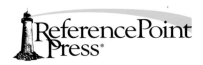

© 2012 ReferencePoint Press, Inc.
Printed in the United States

For more information, contact:
ReferencePoint Press, Inc.
PO Box 27779
San Diego, CA 92198
www.ReferencePointPress.com

Picture credits:
Cover: Dreamstime and iStockphoto.com
Maury Aaseng: 31–34, 46–48, 60–61, 74–76
Dr. Harout Tanielian/Science Photo Library: 11
Thinkstock/iStockphoto.com: 16

LIBRARY OF CONGRESS CATALOGING-IN-PUBLICATION DATA

Parks, Peggy J., 1951–
  Acne and skin disorders / by Peggy J. Parks.
    p. cm. — (Compact research series)
  Includes bibliographical references and index.
  ISBN-13: 978-1-60152-226-9 (hardback)
  ISBN-10: 1-60152-226-6 (hardback)
  1. Acne—Popular works. 2. Skin—Diseases—Popular works. I. Title.
  RL131.P37   2012
  616.5—dc23
                                                    2011033467

Contents

Foreword

As modern civilization continues to evolve, its ability to create, store, distribute, and access information expands exponentially. The explosion of information from all media continues to increase at a phenomenal rate. By 2020 some experts predict the worldwide information base will double every 73 days. While access to diverse sources of information and perspectives is paramount to any democratic society, information alone cannot help people gain knowledge and understanding. Information must be organized and presented clearly and succinctly in order to be understood. The challenge in the digital age becomes not the creation of information, but how best to sort, organize, enhance, and present information.

ReferencePoint Press developed the *Compact Research* series with this challenge of the information age in mind. More than any other subject area today, researching current issues can yield vast, diverse, and unqualified information that can be intimidating and overwhelming for even the most advanced and motivated researcher. The *Compact Research* series offers a compact, relevant, intelligent, and conveniently organized collection of information covering a variety of current topics ranging from illegal immigration and deforestation to diseases such as anorexia and meningitis.

The series focuses on three types of information: objective single-author narratives, opinion-based primary source quotations, and facts and statistics. The clearly written objective narratives provide context and reliable background information. Primary source quotes are carefully selected and cited, exposing the reader to differing points of view. And facts and statistics sections aid the reader in evaluating perspectives. Presenting these key types of information creates a richer, more balanced learning experience.

For better understanding and convenience, the series enhances information by organizing it into narrower topics and adding design features that make it easy for a reader to identify desired content. For example, in *Compact Research: Illegal Immigration*, a chapter covering the economic impact of illegal immigration has an objective narrative explaining the various ways the economy is impacted, a balanced section of numerous primary source quotes on the topic, followed by facts and full-color illustrations to encourage evaluation of contrasting perspectives.

The ancient Roman philosopher Lucius Annaeus Seneca wrote, "It is quality rather than quantity that matters." More than just a collection of content, the *Compact Research* series is simply committed to creating, finding, organizing, and presenting the most relevant and appropriate amount of information on a current topic in a user-friendly style that invites, intrigues, and fosters understanding.

Acne and Skin Disorders at a Glance

Acne Defined

Acne is a disorder of the skin's sebaceous (oil-producing) glands that results in clogged pores and pimples or lesions on the face and other parts of the body.

Prevalence

The National Institutes of Health (NIH) estimates that acne affects nearly 17 million people in the United States, making it one of the most common skin disorders.

Common Skin Disorders

Some of the other most common skin disorders include psoriasis, rosacea, dermatitis, scabies, ringworm, jock itch, and athlete's foot.

Skin Cancer

The three main types of skin cancer are basal cell carcinoma, squamous cell carcinoma, and melanoma. About 2 million Americans are diagnosed with some form of skin cancer each year.

Causes of Acne and Other Skin Disorders

Genetics and hormonal changes may contribute to acne. Genetics, immune system dysfunction, viruses, and infections resulting from fungi or parasites may contribute to or cause other skin disorders.

Ultraviolet Radiation (UV)

Overexposure to UV radiation from sunlight and from artificial tanning devices has been closely connected with premature aging of the skin and skin cancer.

Treatment of Acne and Skin Disorders

Many treatments are available that help keep acne under control. The same is true for other skin disorders, although treatments vary depending on the specific disorder, its severity, and other factors.

Prevention

Limiting exposure to UV radiation can help prevent many cases of skin cancer. Acne, psoriasis, rosacea, and many other skin disorders cannot be prevented, but steps can be taken to keep the disorders under control and, in some cases, to avoid outbreaks.

Overview

❝Acne is the scourge of youth. If you had it, you know exactly how miserable it felt to have all those little red and white bumps and scars on your face, and how helpless you were to prevent them.❞

—Manny Alvarez, chair of the Department of Obstetrics and Gynecology and Reproductive Science at New Jersey's Hackensack University Medical Center and managing editor of health news at FOX News.

❝Because the skin is subjected to many influences and plays a big part in your overall health and well-being, there are many kinds of skin problems. Most can be healed or managed fairly easily.❞

—Palo Alto Medical Foundation, which specializes in medical care, biomedical research, and education.

A s a teenager Lucy Speed considered herself fortunate to have a glowing, unblemished complexion. The British actress remembers how her friends "would moan about their spotty skin" while she "sailed through without so much as a pimple or blocked pore."[1] But to Speed's dismay, the end of her teenage years also marked the end of her flawless skin. By the time she was 20 she had developed a severe case of acne, with skin that was peppered with angry red blemishes. "Friends joked that I was having a second childhood and that the spots made me look younger," she says, "but adult acne is no laughing matter. It's unpleasant at any stage in life but when you are way past puberty it can have a real psychological impact." Speed became distraught over the condition that she felt was ruining her appearance. "The state of my skin affected my personality," she says, "and it has nothing to do with vanity. I became depressed and embarrassed. On a bad day I was full of self-pity and despair."[2]

Speed's struggle with acne dragged on for 10 years. She tried everything, from changing her diet to spending thousands of dollars on skin remedies. Even laser and acupuncture treatments did nothing to clear up her skin. Finally, Speed visited a dermatologist in London who prescribed hormones and also treated her with chemical peels designed to break down dead skin cells. When blemishes erupted on her face, the doctor injected them with antibacterial and anti-inflammatory solutions. Amazingly, Speed's skin totally cleared up within six weeks—and for the first time in years she was happy with the image she saw in the mirror. "The fear that my acne will come back is still there," she says, "but I now feel I have enough knowledge to know how to cope. I understand my battle is ongoing but it is one I am determined to win."[3]

The Marvels of Skin

Understanding skin disorders begins with knowing about the various functions performed by skin. The largest organ in the body, skin holds vital chemicals and nutrients in, while serving as a barrier that keeps dangerous substances out. Acne.com, a website created by a team of dermatologists, explains: "It literally acts as body armor, protecting you from the sun, wind and rain among other environmental factors. As your skin renews itself, it sloughs off dead skin cells to make room for new ones. The process is ongoing and your skin and all its cells are changing continuously."[4]

> **As tough and protective as skin is, it is still vulnerable to a variety of problems.**

Skin has three layers: the epidermis, dermis, and subcutaneous fat. The epidermis (outer layer) is thinner than a piece of plastic wrap, but it is tough and waterproof. An important function of the epidermis is to act as a shield against bacteria, viruses, and other foreign substances and to protect internal organs, muscles, and nerves. Beneath the epidermis is the dermis, which is a thick layer of tissue made up mostly of fibrous proteins known as collagen. Physician and health educator Bernadine Healy writes: "Suffused with collagen, the dermis brings firmness—and when collagen is broken down, wrinkles and sags."[5] The subcutaneous fat layer, which is beneath the dermis, helps to insulate the body from heat and cold, provides protective padding, and softens skin texture.

What Are Acne and Skin Disorders?

As tough and protective as skin is, it is still vulnerable to a variety of problems. Acne, for instance, results from clogged oil glands (known as sebaceous glands), which are located in the dermis and secrete an oily substance called sebum. The NIH writes:

> The oils travel up a canal called a follicle, which also contains a hair. The oils empty onto the skin surface through the follicle's opening, or pore. The hair, oil and cells that line the narrow follicle can form a plug and block the pore, preventing oil from reaching the skin's surface. This mix of oil and cells allows bacteria that normally live on the skin to grow in plugged follicles. Your body's defense system then moves to attack the bacteria and the area gets inflamed. If the plugged follicle stays beneath the skin, you get a white bump called a whitehead. If it reaches the surface of the skin and opens up, you get a blackhead.[6]

The skin disorder known as psoriasis is characterized by a buildup of excess skin tissue on various parts of the body, including the arms, legs, chest, and back. The skin looks red and thick and is often covered with silvery scales. According to Ellen Marmur, chief of the Division of Dermatologic and Cosmetic Surgery at New York City's Mount Sinai Medical Center, psoriasis often causes sufferers extreme distress because of how it affects their appearance. It can also be life-threatening, as she explains: "Not only can it be debilitating socially and emotionally, but people with psoriasis also have a risk of other internal diseases. It's like running your car at maximum, you're just going to burn out the engine and other things are going to go wrong."[7]

Rosacea is typically not as disfiguring as psoriasis, but it can also be traumatic for those who suffer from it. Ted Grossbart, a Harvard Medical School psychologist who specializes in the emotional impact of skin diseases, explains: "Because rosacea affects the way we look, its conse-

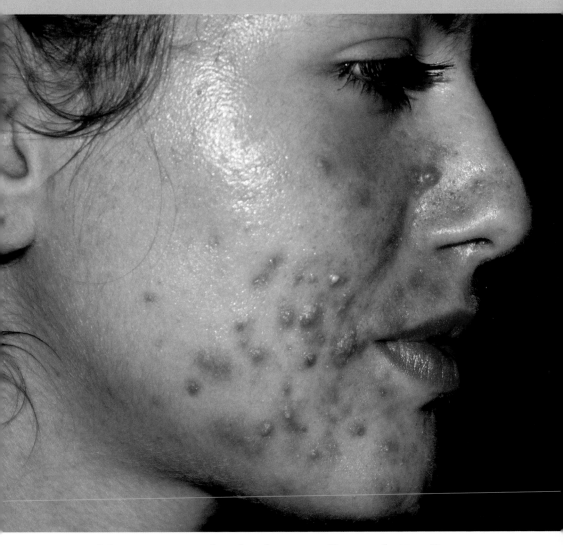

One of the most common skin disorders, acne affects nearly 17 million people in the United States. Hormonal changes may contribute to acne, which explains why many people develop acne during their teenage years.

quences often go far deeper than its physical impact alone. Nobody likes feeling unattractive, and the effect of rosacea on appearance makes a person emotionally vulnerable."[8] Common symptoms of rosacea include flushed skin with pimple-like bumps; tiny, broken blood vessels; watery or bloodshot eyes; and facial burning, stinging, and/or itching. If not treated, rosacea can spread beyond the face to the neck, chest, scalp, ears, or other areas of the body.

Itching, Oozing, and Crusting

Dermatitis (also known as eczema) is an umbrella term for inflammation of the skin that usually involves swelling, redness, and itchiness. One of the most common types is contact dermatitis, which is so named because it results from direct contact with an allergen (such as soaps, chemicals, or metals) or an irritant like poison ivy, oak, or sumac. These weeds contain a sap called urushiol, which escapes from damaged areas of a plant. People can be exposed to urushiol at any time of the year by touching the plants, having contact with an object that has become contaminated, or being exposed to airborne particles from lawn mowing or burning.

> One of the most common types is contact dermatitis, which is so named because it results from direct contact with an allergen (such as soaps, chemicals, or metals) or an irritant like poison ivy, oak, or sumac.

Even more common is atopic dermatitis, which involves inflammation in the upper layers of the skin. Anyone can develop it, but it is most prevalent among children: An estimated 10 to 20 percent of children suffer from it, compared with 1 to 3 percent of adults. According to Princeton University Health Services, people with atopic dermatitis have an overactive inflammatory response to irritating substances (or triggers), which causes their skin to itch. "Triggers vary," the group explains, "but may include rough or coarse materials, detergents, soaps, juices from fruit and meats, dust mites, and animal saliva and dander. Some people break out in rash when feeling too hot and/or sweaty. The rash typically arises on the face, neck, and the insides of elbows, knees, and ankles."[9]

Cancers of the Skin

Skin cancer is the most common type of cancer in the United States. According to the American Academy of Dermatology (AAD), an estimated 2 million Americans are diagnosed with some form of it each year, and 1 out of 5 will develop it in their lifetimes. Skin cancer is divided into two main groups: nonmelanoma, which includes basal cell carcinoma and squamous cell carcinoma, and melanoma. Basal cell carcinoma is the most common type and begins in basal cells, or skin cells, which produce new cells as old ones die. Squamous cell carcinoma originates in squamous cells, which are flat, thin cells that make up the outer layer of the skin. This type of skin cancer often appears as nodules or red, scaly patches, and unlike basal cell carcinoma, it can spread to other parts of the body.

Melanoma develops in the cells that produce melanin, the pigment that gives skin its color, and is the rarest of all skin cancers—as well as the deadliest. Studies have shown that melanoma represents only 3 percent of skin cancer cases but is responsible

> " Melanoma develops in the cells that produce melanin, the pigment that gives skin its color, and is the rarest of all skin cancers—as well as the deadliest. "

for 75 percent of all skin cancer deaths. The most common symptom is changes in the skin, especially to moles. The American Skin Association says that these changes may involve moles that start bleeding or crusting; borders that become irregular or jagged; and moles that are odd shaped, such as one half not matching the other. Another warning sign is changing color, as the group explains: "The majority of melanomas are black or brown. However, some melanomas are skin-colored, pink, red, purple blue or white."[10]

Not Just for Teenagers

Acne is most common among adolescents, but it can develop at any age. People in their forties and fifties can develop acne, as can young children. Even babies can get acne, as physicians from Seton Healthcare in Austin, Texas, write: "It isn't just teens who are affected by acne. Sometimes newborns have acne because their mothers pass hormones to them just before delivery. Acne can also appear when the stress of birth causes the baby's body to release hormones on its own."[11]

Acne that does not clear up by about the age of 20 is referred to as persistent acne, whereas late-onset acne develops after the age of 21.

As was the case with Speed, late-onset acne can be perplexing and distressing for those who develop it. The AAD writes: "People who have not had acne for years can suddenly see deep-seated, inflamed pimples and nodules. Even those who have never had acne get late-onset acne."[12] According to Tampa, Florida, dermatologist Robert A. Norman, men who develop acne tend to have more severe, longer-lasting types, whereas women typically experience flare-ups at times of hormonal shifts, such as during their menstrual cycles.

What Causes Acne and Skin Disorders?

Although scientists are not certain what causes acne, hormones have been shown to play a major role in its development. This is why it is more common during puberty, as well as the reason women tend to break out before their menstrual periods. Physician and FOX News health news editor Manny Alvarez writes: "Other than the role of hormones, and in particular the male hormone, androgen, the exact cause of acne is not known. During puberty there is an increase in the androgen hormone in both boys and in girls, causing the oil glands to enlarge and produce more oil."[13]

> Contrary to its name, ringworm has nothing to do with worms; rather, it is so named because the infection causes ring-shaped patches on the face, head, trunk, arms, legs, or scalp.

A number of skin conditions develop because of infections from parasites or fungi. Scabies, for instance, results from infestation by an eight-legged itch mite called *Sarcoptes scabiei*. Physician James G.H. Dinulos explains: "The female itch mite tunnels in the topmost layer of the skin and deposits her eggs in burrows. Young mites (larvae) then hatch in a few days. The infestation causes intense itching, probably from an allergic reaction to the mites."[14] Dinulos adds that scabies spreads easily from person to person on physical contact.

Two skin disorders that are caused by fungi are ringworm and jock itch. Contrary to its name, ringworm has nothing to do with worms; rather, it is so named because the infection causes ring-shaped patches on the face, head, trunk, arms, legs, or scalp. The fungal skin disorder jock itch, which usually affects adult men and adolescent boys, is an infection of the groin area and develops when fungus grows and multiplies. According to the NIH, jock itch can be triggered by friction from clothes and prolonged wetness from sweating, which is why the skin disorder is common among athletes.

Effects of Sunlight

The sun makes all life on earth possible, and no living thing could survive without it. One of the sun's innumerable benefits is that its ultraviolet (UV) rays help the body produce vitamin D, an essential nutrient that is often called the "sunshine" vitamin. Vitamin D helps protect against diseases such as rickets, which leads to softening and weakening of the bones. Yet only a small amount of sunlight is necessary for the production of vitamin D—as little as 10 minutes a day, according to the Mayo Clinic—and too much UV exposure can be harmful. The rays known as UVB penetrate the top layers of skin and are most responsible for sunburns, while UVA rays penetrate to the deeper layers of the skin. Both kinds of UV rays can cause thinning of the epidermis and dermis, which leads to premature aging of the skin, as well as the development of wrinkles.

> " **Both kinds of UV rays can cause thinning of the epidermis and dermis, which leads to premature aging of the skin, as well as the development of wrinkles.** "

By far, though, the greatest risk of overexposure to UV radiation is skin cancer. The US Department of Health and Human Services and the World Health Organization have identified UV radiation as a proven human carcinogen. In fact, UV radiation is considered the number one cause of nonmelanoma skin cancers and a leading cause of melanoma—and this includes not only UV light from the sun, but also from artificial tanning beds. The Skin Cancer Foundation explains: "The high-pressure sunlamps used in tanning salons emit doses of UVA as much as 12 times that of the sun. Not surprisingly, people who use tanning salons are 2.5

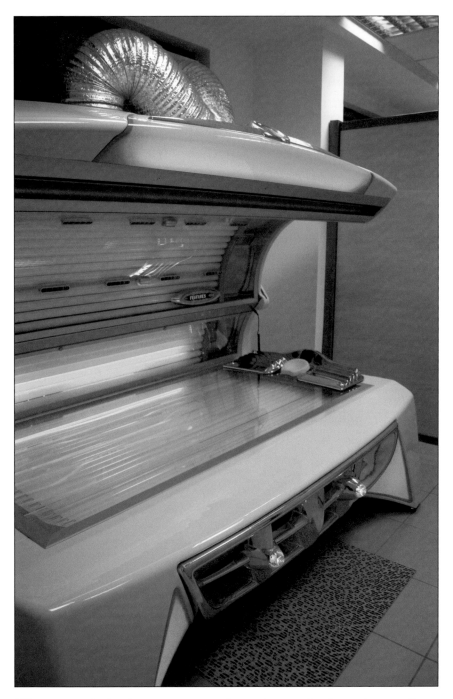

The tanning bed industry sometimes claims that artificial tanning is safer than natural sunlight, but research has shown this to be false. People who use tanning beds (pictured) have a heightened risk of developing skin cancer.

times more likely to develop squamous cell carcinoma, and 1.5 times more likely to develop basal cell carcinoma."[15]

Diagnosing Acne and Skin Disorders

Different procedures are used to diagnose skin disorders, depending on the nature of the condition. In many cases, dermatologists can identify the disorders (including acne) just by examining the skin. Physician Robert J. MacNeal explains: "Revealing characteristics include size, shape, color, and location of the abnormality as well as the presence or absence of other symptoms or signs."[16] When fungal or parasitic infections are suspected, doctors scrape off a small amount of material from the skin and examine it under a microscope or test it in a laboratory culture.

As with all types of cancer, skin cancer is diagnosed through biopsy, which involves numbing a small area of skin and cutting out all or part of a suspicious mole or other lesion. The sample is then analyzed by a pathologist. If the diagnosis of skin cancer is confirmed, the next step is for the physician to determine the extent (stage) of the cancer and whether it has spread. Regarding melanoma, the Mayo Clinic writes: "Melanoma is staged using the Roman numerals I through IV. A stage I melanoma is small and has a very successful treatment rate. But the higher the numeral, the lower the chances of a full recovery. By stage IV, the cancer has spread beyond your skin to other organs, such as your lungs or liver."[17]

How Are Acne and Skin Disorders Treated?

Numerous treatments are available for acne, and if caught early enough, it can often be brought under control. Alvarez writes: "All the medications available for acne basically attempt to decrease the oil production, the inflammation, and any secondary infection caused when bacteria is trapped under the skin."[18] Mild to moderate acne is typically treated with topical (meaning applied directly to the skin) creams or lotions that contain benzoyl peroxide or salicylic acid. More severe cases may be treated with tretinoin (brand names include Retin-A), a drug derived from vitamin A, and/or other prescription drugs given by mouth or injection.

Other types of skin disorder treatments are prescribed based on the individual condition and its severity. Dermatologists often treat rosacea with a combination of topical and oral drugs. Patients are given antibiotics (such as tetracycline) by mouth, as well as creams or gels that are

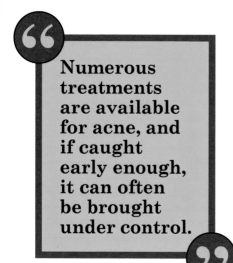

> Numerous treatments are available for acne, and if caught early enough, it can often be brought under control.

rubbed on the skin to help relieve symptoms. Fungal infections such as ringworm or jock itch are treated with oral and/or topical antifungal medications.

By its very nature, skin cancer involves more complex treatment than what is typically prescribed for other skin disorders—and time is of the essence. According to the AAD, skin cancers, including melanoma, have cure rates of nearly 100 percent if they are caught and treated early enough. The cancerous growth is often removed through a surgical procedure known as excision, whereby the dermatologist numbs the skin and then cuts out (excises) the cancerous growth. A small amount of skin that does not show signs of cancer may also be excised so the doctor can determine whether cancer cells are still present in the skin.

Can Acne and Skin Disorders Be Prevented?

Although acne is not actually a preventable skin disorder, dermatologists say that diligent skin care can help prevent it or keep it under control if breakouts occur. The AAD recommends washing the skin twice a day with mild soap and warm water, but warns against vigorous washing and scrubbing that could cause irritation and make the acne worse. New York dermatologist Diane S. Berson explains: "Harsh cleansers, alkaline bar soaps and alcohol-based products may worsen irritation. Cleansing products with mild surfactants can remove surface oil and dirt without compromising the skin's barrier function."[19]

One skin disorder that is highly preventable is skin cancer. Because of its close connection with UV radiation, people who diligently apply sunscreen, avoid long-term exposure to the sun, and wear protective clothing when they are in the sun vastly reduce their skin cancer risk. The AAD writes: "Sun exposure is the most preventable risk factor for all skin cancers, including melanoma. You can have fun in the sun and decrease your risk of skin cancer."[20] Equally important, according to the AAD, the Skin Cancer Foundation, and other health organizations, is avoiding the use of artificial tanning devices.

Tough, Yet Vulnerable

Skin is an amazing organ, one that shields and protects the body in numerous ways. But it is also vulnerable to a wide variety of disorders, from acne to skin cancer. Many skin problems can be successfully treated, and some can be cured. Whether they are preventable or not depends on the nature of the disorder and the root of its cause.

What Are Acne and Skin Disorders?

66Acne. Zits. Pimples. Blemishes. No matter what you call them, acne can be distressing and annoyingly persistent.99

—Mayo Clinic, a world-renowned medical facility headquartered in Rochester, Minnesota.

66People with skin problems are at high risk of developing psychological problems, and they can linger even after the skin gets better.99

—Ted Grossbart, a psychologist with Harvard Medical School and author of the book *Skin Deep: A Mind/Body Approach to Healthy Skin*.

Seppo Puusa, a young man from Finland, developed his first pimple when he was 15 years old, and that marked the beginning of a struggle with acne that lasted for more than a decade. He says that at first he was not too concerned about it. "Until one day I got a huge pimple on the tip of my nose. It was one of those couldn't be bigger, couldn't be any redder and couldn't be in a worse spot pimples; think Rudolph the Reindeer, and you'll get the idea."[21] When a friend cracked a joke about the pimple, that was when the acne really started to bother Puusa—and before long, his acne grew worse. He writes:

> During the last years of high school I developed a massive, that's the only word to describe it, back acne. My entire

20

back was covered in huge cysts. Luckily Finland is not much of a beach country (too cold for that), but sauna plays a big part in our social life. . . . You can imagine that my back acne didn't make those events easy. I was often the only one wearing a t-shirt or huddled in a corner.[22]

Over the following years Puusa tried every possible remedy, from creams, lotions, and ointments to antibiotics. He thought he had finally found the answer in a prescription drug called Accutane, which cleared up his skin within two months. His happiness was short-lived, however. Even though his back acne did not return, he developed a severe case of acne on his scalp. "That was the only permanent effect Accutane had," he says. "Now I had a scalp full of pimples. I guess you could call that progress; at least it was less visible. But it didn't make me enthusiastic about getting [a] haircut."[23]

Scarred Sufferers

Although millions of people young and old struggle with acne, its effects vary widely from person to person. Manny Alvarez writes: "A field guide of acne lesions would include everything from *pustules*, or simple pimples, to *papules*, or small pink bumps on the skin that are tender to the touch, to very large *nodules*, which are painful solid lesions locked deep in the skin, to *cysts*, those deep, painful, pus-filled lesions that can cause scarring."[24] Not everyone with acne sustains the tissue damage that causes permanent scars on the skin. But even those who are not physically scarred often suffer emotionally because of how the skin disorder affects their appearance.

According to the AAD, research has shown that severe or long-lasting acne can result in deep insecurity that can last throughout someone's

> " Not everyone with acne sustains the tissue damage that causes permanent scars on the skin. But even those who are not physically scarred often suffer emotionally because of how the skin disorder affects their appearance. "

lifetime. The group explains: "One study found that people who had acne for a significant amount of time tend to feel 'scarred for life.' Long after the acne clears, they may have low self-esteem and feelings of in-feriority." The AAD adds that anxiety and low self-esteem are common among people with severe acne, and even those with mild to moderate cases often suffer from psychological distress. "When asked to talk about how acne affects them," says the AAD, "patients often mention feelings of inferiority, embarrassment, and depression. One teenager said, 'I was more self-conscious about my skin, and at times very shy because I felt my acne made me very ugly.'"[25]

> The effects of psoriasis go far beyond bumps or pimples. Large swaths of skin on the face, arms, hands, and legs become thickened and bright red, splotched with raw, scaly patches that often crack open and bleed.

The emotional turmoil that accompanies acne was the focus of a study published in September 2010 by researchers from Norway. Nearly 3,800 teenagers were involved in the study, of which 14 percent said they suffered from either moderate or severe acne. The research team found that the teens with the worst cases were far more likely to have few friends and poor grades in school than those with clear skin. Even more disturbing was an elevated suicide risk among the teens with severe acne. Nearly 25 percent said they had considered suicide, compared with 11 percent of the study participants overall. Psychologist John Grohol writes: "So the latest finding confirms what we already know about acne—it's a debilitating condition for those who suffer [from] it. So debilitating that it appears to be significantly correlated with suicidal thoughts and depression."[26]

The Utter Misery of Psoriasis

Anyone who has a severe skin disorder is well aware of how traumatic it can be—and for many with psoriasis, emotional trauma is a constant companion. The effects of psoriasis go far beyond bumps or pimples. Large swaths of skin on the face, arms, hands, and legs become thickened and bright red, splotched with raw, scaly patches that often crack open and bleed. Such disfiguring changes in their appearance causes sufferers to feel a deep sense of shame and embarrassment, as model CariDee English explains: "It's a battle. . . . You feel icky, ugly and insecure—and ostracized, like you're the only one who has it."[27]

English was just two years old when she was diagnosed with psoriasis. As a young girl she dreamed of someday becoming a model, but her family tried to dissuade her because of the severity of her skin condition. "It was difficult for anyone to take me seriously," she says. "My family—God bless them—tried to protect me by saying that I had to choose another career."[28] In 2006 English seemed to have beaten the odds by landing a coveted spot on the television program *America's Next Top Model*, and her lifelong dream came true when she was chosen as the winner. But her struggle with psoriasis was far from over. In September 2009 she suffered her worst attack ever, an outbreak so severe that she had to stop working to focus on treatment: "It was horrible—70% of my skin from head to toe was covered in psoriasis, and it was the first time my hands were totally covered in it."[29]

English found a dermatologist who specializes in psoriasis, and he developed a treatment plan that eventually cleared up her skin. But before starting the regimen, she made a courageous decision. Rather than go into hiding until she was no longer covered in angry red blotches, she posed for photographs that revealed the severity of her disorder. She explains: "I wanted to make it a source of empowerment. Before I started the new medication, I thought, 'How can I best utilize this flare-up to help other people?' I decided I would document myself fully exposed, with the hope that if a girl can see that out in the open, it can give them hope there's something concrete out there that can help them."[30]

> "According to recent news reports, another plant that causes skin reactions has been found in Canada and the United States—but its effects are much more hazardous than irritation and itchiness."

Nightmare Weeds

One of the most common skin disorders is contact dermatitis, especially the type that involves allergies to poison ivy, oak, and/or sumac. According to Princeton University Health Services, up to 85 percent of the population is sensitive to urushiol, the sap of these weeds. The group writes: "Affected areas will initially itch, and then become red, swollen, and blistered. In severe cases, patients develop oozing sores."[31] According to recent news reports, another plant that causes skin reactions has been found in Canada and the United States—but its effects are much more hazardous than irritation and itchiness.

A native of Central Asia, *Heracleum mantegazzianum* (commonly known as giant hogweed) has been found in a number of New England states, as well as in Michigan, Ohio, Washington, and Oregon. According to health officials, it is spreading rapidly, especially in the state of New York, where sightings of the plant soared between 2010 and 2011. The giant hogweed can reach heights of up to 20 feet (6.1m), and its clusters of white flowers are as big as umbrellas. When exposed to sunlight, the plant's clear, watery sap bonds with human skin, causing a dangerous chemical reaction. Forestry official Jeff Muzzi, who has been investigating giant hogweed sightings in Canada, explains: "What it does to you is pretty ugly. It causes blisters. Large blisters and permanent scarring. What's left over looks like a scar from a chemical burn or fire."[32]

By far the greatest risk posed by giant hogweed is to the eyes. According to Muzzi, if even a tiny trace of the sap gets into someone's eye, it can burn the cornea and cause temporary or permanent blindness. Several states have reported that children who broke off the plant's large, hollow stems and used them as pretend telescopes were blinded when the toxic sap got into their eyes.

Nonmelanoma Skin Cancers

Skin cancer is a diagnosis that no one wants to hear. But those who have basal cell or squamous cell carcinoma can take comfort in knowing that these skin cancers are highly curable, as Princeton University Health Services writes: "They are superficial, slow-growing, and easily treatable if caught early."[33] Some of the risk factors for nonmelanoma skin cancers include light-colored skin, blue or green eyes, and blond or red hair. Both basal cell and squamous cell carcinoma develop most often on skin that is regularly exposed to UV radiation from the sun or from artificial tanning devices.

Basal cell carcinoma starts in the epidermis and often appears as a new skin growth that bleeds easily and/or does not heal. According to the NIH, this type of skin cancer grows very slowly and almost never spreads beyond the skin. Says the NIH: "Basal cell skin cancer used to be more common in people over age 40, but is now often diagnosed in younger people."[34]

Squamous cell carcinoma, which most often affects people over the age of 50, develops when something causes skin cells to change, such as when skin has been injured or becomes inflamed. The NIH says that the main symptom is a "growing bump that may have a rough, scaly surface and flat reddish patches. The bump is usually located on the face, ears, neck, hands, or arms, but may occur on other areas."[35] The NIH adds that squamous cell carcinoma cancer grows faster than the basal cell type, and while it can spread to other areas of the body, it rarely does.

> " Skin cancer is a diagnosis that no one wants to hear. But those who have basal cell or squamous cell carcinoma can take comfort in knowing that these skin cancers are highly curable. "

"A Vicious, Nasty Disease"

Melanoma is characterized by the uncontrolled growth of pigment-producing skin cells known as melanocytes. According to the AAD, melanoma is the most common form of cancer for young adults aged 25 to 29 and the second-most-common cancer for adolescents and young adults aged 15 to 29. Like nonmelanoma skin cancers, melanoma is treatable if caught in the earliest stages. But because it affects deeper layers of the skin than other skin cancers and is extremely aggressive, it has the greatest potential to spread rapidly to the lymph nodes and other organs. For those reasons melanoma is the most dangerous type of skin cancer, accounting for 75 percent of all skin cancer deaths. According to the Skin Cancer Foundation, the survival rate for patients whose melanoma is detected early (before the cancerous growth has penetrated the skin) is about 99 percent—and plummets to 15 percent or less for those in advanced stages.

One melanoma victim was Nicole Lariviere, a 33-year-old elementary school psychologist from Colorado. In January 2009 Lariviere had a routine physical, and the doctor recommended that a mole on her skin be removed and biopsied. Tests showed that she had melanoma. The doctor removed additional skin around the mole, and Lariviere thought the procedure had taken care of the problem. That summer she returned to the doctor for a 6-month checkup, and a chest X-ray showed that the cancer had spread to her lungs. Within a few months it spread beyond the lungs into her ovaries, pancreas, abdomen, and brain. The day after Thanksgiving 2009—less than a year after the mole tested positive for melanoma—the aggressive cancer claimed Lariviere's life. Friend and colleague Jessica McMichael shares her thoughts: "People think melanoma and they think, 'Oh, just go and have it cut off and you're good,' but it's a vicious, nasty disease."[36]

An Array of Problems

From acne to dermatitis, psoriasis, and skin cancer, millions of people suffer from disorders of the skin. Some of these are relatively minor and clear up either on their own or with treatment. Others, however, result in drastic changes in appearance that cause emotional trauma—and in some cases, such as with melanoma, can be deadly.

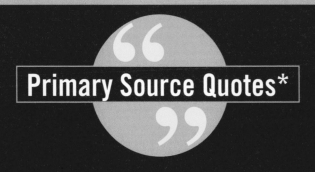

Primary Source Quotes*

What Are Acne and Skin Disorders?

66 How serious is acne? It's certainly not life-threatening; you won't die from acne. But it is a serious matter, especially for those who suffer from it. 99

—Melanie Vasseur, *Under My Skin*. Campbell, CA: FastPencil, 2010.

Vasseur is a nutritional cosmetic chemist and medical esthetician from San Diego, California.

66 Basal cell cancers appear as pearly or waxy nodules with central depressions or craters. As this cancer enlarges, the center usually becomes more ulcerated, giving it the appearance of having been gnawed. 99

—James M. Fries and Donald M. Vickery, *Take Care of Yourself*. Cambridge, MA: Da Capo, 2009.

Fries is a professor of medicine at Stanford University, and Vickery was head of the nonprofit Self-Care Institute before his death in 2008.

* Editor's Note: While the definition of a primary source can be narrowly or broadly defined, for the purposes of Compact Research, a primary source consists of: 1) results of original research presented by an organization or researcher; 2) eyewitness accounts of events, personal experience, or work experience; 3) first-person editorials offering pundits' opinions; 4) government officials presenting political plans and/or policies; 5) representatives of organizations presenting testimony or policy.

66 **Eczema is a general term for any type of dermatitis or 'itchy rash.' . . . All types of eczemas cause itching and redness and some will blister, weep or peel.** 99

—National Eczema Association, "Eczema Quick Fact Sheet," July 10, 2011. www.nationaleczema.org.

Through research, support, and education, the National Eczema Association seeks to improve the health and quality of life for people with eczema.

66 **Acne manifests in an amazingly complex range of symptoms. It is complicated by stress, hormonal changes, and other health issues.** 99

—Ava Shamban, *Heal Your Skin*. Hoboken, NJ: Wiley, 2011.

Shamban is a dermatologist from Santa Monica, California, and the dermatology expert for the television series *Extreme Makeover*.

66 **In atopic dermatitis, the skin becomes extremely itchy. Scratching leads to redness, swelling, cracking, 'weeping' clear fluid, and finally, crusting and scaling.** 99

—National Institute of Arthritis and Musculoskeletal and Skin Diseases, "Atopic Dermatitis," May 2009. www.niams.nih.gov.

The institute supports research into the causes, treatment, and prevention of arthritis and musculoskeletal and skin diseases, trains scientists to carry out this research, and provides information on research progress.

66 **Recent studies have questioned whether there truly is a melanoma epidemic or if rising rates reflect a change in how doctors diagnose melanoma and the availability of skin cancer screenings.** 99

—AAD, "Melanoma Trends," 2011. www.aad.org.

Composed of over 17,000 dermatologists, the AAD is dedicated to education, research, and patient advocacy.

❝People sometimes call rosacea 'adult acne' because it can cause outbreaks that look like acne. It can also cause burning and soreness in the eyes and eyelids.❞

—Palo Alto Medical Foundation, "Rosacea," August 12, 2010. www.pamf.org.

The Palo Alto Medical Foundation specializes in medical care, biomedical research, and education.

....

❝In addition to cosmetic effects, which can include permanent scarring, acne can have detrimental effects on self-image and social interactions.❞

—Christine Laine and David R. Goldmann, *In the Clinic: Practical Information About Common Health Problems.* Philadelphia: ACP, 2009.

Laine and Goldmann are internal medicine physicians from Philadelphia, Pennsylvania.

....

❝Because psoriasis is misunderstood and literally covered up by clothing, people with psoriasis are often subjected to discrimination at work, in spas and pools and in salons.❞

—Paul Yamauchi, interviewed by *Skincare News*, "Psoriasis Expert Dr. Paul Yamauchi Talks About Treating Chronic Skin Conditions," SkinCare-News.com, April 19, 2010. www.skincare-news.com.

Yamauchi is a dermatologist and the medical director of the Dermatology Institute & Skin Care Center of Santa Monica, California.

....

Facts and Illustrations

What Are Acne and Skin Disorders?

- According to the Pharmaceutical Research and Manufacturers of America, more than **100 million** people in the United States (one-third of the US population) are afflicted with skin disorders.

- The AAD states that over **3.5 million** skin cancers in more than **2 million** people are diagnosed each year in the United States.

- According to the Centers for Disease Control and Prevention, **8 out of 10** preteens and teens develop some form of acne.

- A study published in August 2010 by researchers from China found that **52.74 percent** of male Chinese adolescents and **49.65 percent** of female Chinese adolescents suffer from acne.

- According to health officials in Spain, melanoma cases rose **7 percent** between 2010 and 2011.

- A study published in the August 2010 issue of the *Journal of Investigative Dermatology* found that prevalence of eczema among children in the United States ranged from **8.7 to 18.1 percent**, with the highest prevalence reported in many East Coast states, as well as in Nevada, Utah, and Idaho.

- A study published in 2010 by researchers from the United Kingdom found that the rates of men dying from **melanoma** have doubled since the 1970s.

Most Common Skin Disorders

A report published in June 2011 by the Pharmaceutical Research and Manufacturers of America states that over 100 million people in the United States are afflicted with skin disorders, of which actinic keratoses (precancerous skin growths) are the most common. This graph shows the estimated prevalence of five of the most common skin disorders.

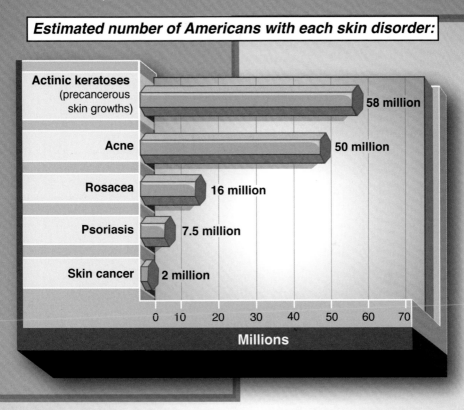

Estimated number of Americans with each skin disorder:

Disorder	Millions
Actinic keratoses (precancerous skin growths)	58 million
Acne	50 million
Rosacea	16 million
Psoriasis	7.5 million
Skin cancer	2 million

Source: Pharmaceutical Research and Manufacturers of America, "Biopharmaceutical Research Companies Are Developing 300 Medicines to Treat Diseases of the Skin," *Medicines in Development for Skin Diseases*, June 2011. www.phrma.org.

- The World Health Organization estimates that over **2 million** cases of skin cancer, including an estimated **132,000** cases of malignant melanoma, occur worldwide each year.

- According to the Skin Cancer Foundation, an estimated **13 million** people in the United States are living with either basal cell or squamous cell carcinoma.

The Emotional Trauma of Psoriasis

Psoriasis is one of the most disfiguring skin disorders, causing large swaths of skin to thicken and turn bright red and scaly. A study published in August 2010 found that people who suffer from severe psoriasis have a markedly increased risk of depression, anxiety, and suicidal thoughts.

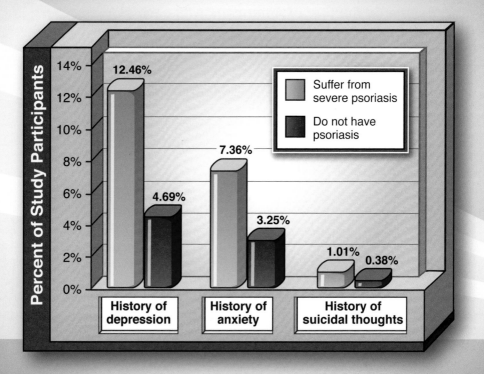

Source: Shanu Kohli Kurd et al. "The Risk of Depression, Anxiety, and Suicidality in Patients with Psoriasis," *Archives of Dermatology*, August 2010. http://archderm.ama-assn.org.

- The NIH states that about **80 percent** of people between the ages of 11 and 30 have outbreaks of the skin at some point in their lives.

- According to the National Cancer Institute, melanoma represents only **3 percent** of skin cancer cases but is responsible for **75 percent** of all skin cancer deaths.

Melanoma Is the Deadliest Skin Cancer

According to the American Cancer Society, melanoma accounts for less than 5 percent of all skin cancer cases, but it causes an estimated 75 percent of deaths from skin cancer. These graphs show the prevalence and mortality rates of basal cell and squamous cell carcinoma, compared with melanoma.

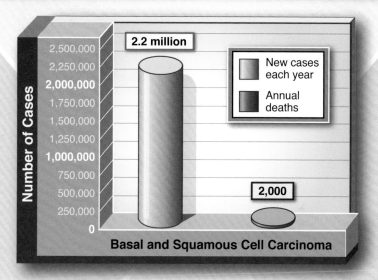

Source: American Cancer Society, "Skin Cancer: Basal and Squamous Cell Carcinoma," May 10, 2011. www.cancer.org.

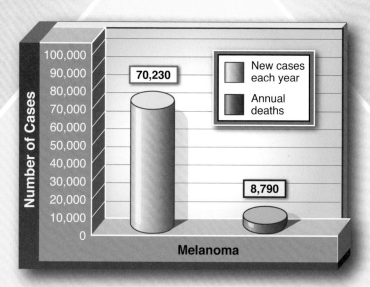

Source: American Cancer Society, "Learn About Cancer: Melanoma Skin Cancer Overview," May 5, 2011. www.cancer.org.

Teens Desperate to Be Acne-Free

During a survey published in March 2011, representatives from the United Kingdom group Acne Academy interviewed more than 500 British teenagers to gauge their perceptions about acne. As this graph shows, the teens suffering from acne are bothered by the skin condition so much that they would willingly give up privileges and make sacrifices in return for getting rid of it.

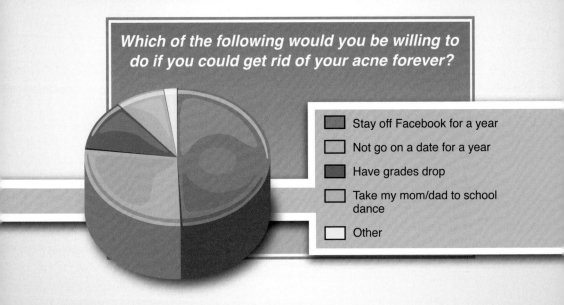

Which of the following would you be willing to do if you could get rid of your acne forever?

- Stay off Facebook for a year
- Not go on a date for a year
- Have grades drop
- Take my mom/dad to school dance
- Other

Source: Acne Academy, *Acne Perceptions*, March 2011. www.acneperceptions.com.

- According to the National Institute of Arthritis and Musculoskel-etal and Skin Diseases, approximately **14 million** people in the United States have rosacea, and it most often affects adults between the ages of 30 and 60.

- The US Environmental Protection Agency states that each year, more new cases of **skin cancer** are diagnosed in the United States than new cases of breast, prostate, lung, and colon cancers combined.

- According to the AAD, from **10 to 50 million** people in the United States have an allergic reaction to poison ivy each year.

What Causes Acne and Skin Disorders?

66There are many myths about what causes acne. Some people blame foods for their outbreaks. Some think that dirty skin causes it. But there's little evidence that either has much effect on most people's acne.99

—NIH, the United States' leading medical research agency.

66Skin problems are multifactorial, like everything else, with genetic predispositions, nutrition factors, hormonal influences, medication side effects, stress factors, inflammatory pathology all playing a role.99

—Julia Tatum Hunter, a dermatologist from Beverly Hills, California.

Joanne Cobb was 15 years old when she used a tanning bed for the first time. She loved the golden glow of her skin and wanted to keep it year-round, so she tanned often. By the time she was 21, she was using a tanning bed (sometimes called a sunbed) 5 times a week, and during the summer months, she spent hours in the sun without worrying about using sunscreen. "I would definitely describe myself as tanorexic," she says. "It reached the point where I would feel panicked every time my tan started to fade." In 2009 Cobb had a doctor check a mole on her leg and found that she had developed melanoma. "I immediately made the connection between the condition and all those years I had spent in the sun," she says. "I vowed there and then never to go on a sunbed again."[37]

Cobb, who has four little boys, wishes she had made that decision years earlier. She has undergone surgery to have lymph nodes removed because the cancer had spread through her bloodstream and into her groin and pelvis. For now doctors have given her the all clear, but they warned that there is a 50 percent chance of the cancer returning within five years—and if it does, it will kill her, as there is nothing more they can do. Every day Cobb lives with the awareness that her sons might lose their mother at a young age, and that is unbearably painful for her. "I just wish I could turn back the clock," she says. "If I hadn't ignored the risks I would never have found myself in this position. I try not to think about it, but the reality is that my life will be a lot shorter thanks to skin cancer."[38]

No Safe Tanning

What happened to Cobb is becoming more and more common, as statistics show that skin cancer is on the rise. According to an April 2010 paper by researchers from California, melanoma incidence is increasing by 2.5 percent annually, and mortality has risen by approximately 44 percent since 1973. Many health officials attribute this spike to the growing popularity of tanning salons. In fact, the International Agency for Research on Cancer includes artificial tanning devices in its list of the most dangerous cancer-causing substances—the same list that includes not only solar UV radiation but also arsenic, plutonium (used to make nuclear weapons), tobacco, and other known carcinogens. Many tanning salon owners, as well as the Indoor Tanning Association, have claimed that artificial tanning is safer than natural sunlight, which the US Food and Drug Administration (FDA) adamantly refutes:

> Advocates of tanning devices sometimes argue that using these devices is less dangerous than sun tanning because the intensity of UV radiation and the time spent tanning can be controlled. But there is no evidence to support these claims. In fact, sunlamps may be more dangerous than the sun because they can be used at the same high intensity every day of the year—unlike the sun whose intensity varies with the time of day, the season, and cloud cover.[39]

A study published in May 2010 confirmed that no tanning device can be considered safe. Conducted by researchers from the University of Minnesota School of Public Health, the study examined the relationship between artificial tanning and skin cancer. It involved 2,268 adults from Minnesota, including 1,167 who had been diagnosed with melanoma between 2004 and 2007 and 1,101 without skin cancer. Based on their findings, the researchers concluded that people who had used any type of artificial tanning device were 74 percent more likely to develop melanoma than those who had not tanned in this way. Lead investigator DeAnn Lazovich explains: "We found that it didn't matter the type of tanning device used; there was no safe tanning device. We also found—and this is new data—that the risk of getting melanoma is associated more with how much a person tans and not the age at which a person starts using tanning devices."[40]

> According to an April 2010 paper by researchers from California, melanoma incidence is increasing by 2.5 percent annually, and mortality has risen by approximately 44 percent since 1973.

Acne's Family Ties

The link between heredity and many skin disorders has long been of interest to scientists. Acne, for instance, is considered to be at least somewhat connected with genes because it is known to run in families. Skin care educator Angela Palmer, who specializes in the treatment of acne and skin problems, writes: "Just like the color of your eyes and the shape of your nose, acne seems to be hereditary. So if Mom or Dad (or both) had acne, it's more likely that you'll develop it too. And the more members of your family with acne, the greater the chances you have of developing the problem."[41]

Examining the role of genetics in the development of acne was the major focus of a 2009 study of teenagers by researchers from Iran and Germany. It involved 1,002 high school students from Tehran, Iran, including 503 girls and 499 boys, who were classified into three groups:

> **One of the study's findings was that a family history of acne was significantly more common among the teens with moderate to severe acne than those who had mild acne.**

no family history of acne (parents, brothers and/or sisters), history in one family member, and history in two or more family members. At the conclusion of the study, the team determined that heredity was the strongest factor among the teens who suffered from acne.

One of the study's findings was that a family history of acne was significantly more common among the teens with moderate to severe acne than those who had mild acne, which the researchers say is consistent with previous research. They also found that a mother with a history of acne most often determined whether a child would go on to develop it, followed by the father, whose acne history was more influential than that of older sisters or brothers. Moreover, the more family members who had acne, the higher the risk for the teens also to develop moderate to severe forms of it.

Genes and Psoriasis

Like acne, psoriasis tends to run in families. According to the National Psoriasis Foundation, if one parent has the disorder, a child has about a 10 percent chance of also developing it. If both parents have it, their children's likelihood of developing it jumps to 50 percent. Although much remains unknown about psoriasis, scientists do know that it is an autoimmune disease, meaning that the immune system produces antibodies against its own tissues. The American Academy of Family Physicians writes: "Your immune system usually protects the body against infection and disease by attacking bacteria and viruses. However, when you have psoriasis, your T cells, a kind of white blood cells that are part of the immune system, mistakenly attack your skin cells instead. Your body then produces other immune system responses, leading to swelling and rapid production of skin cells."[42]

In July 2011 researchers from Germany announced a study that may help clear up the mystery of why the T cells in people with psoriasis malfunction the way they do. The team examined a small group of patients who suffer from both psoriasis and eczema. Through their investigation, the researchers found that the T cells in both skin disorders migrate to the skin in response to environmental triggers, rather than the cells themselves being abnormal. If scientists could now determine the specific triggers that stimulate each condition, this could lead to new ways to stop psoriasis and eczema from developing in people who are genetically predisposed.

The Role of Diet

Many experts contend that a person's diet does not influence whether he or she develops acne, as the AAD writes: "Extensive scientific studies have not found a connection between diet and acne. In other words, food does not cause acne. Not chocolate. Not french fries. Not pizza."[43] This is a controversial viewpoint, however, because some studies suggest that diet *does* play a role in the development of acne. One that was published in 2008 by researchers from the Harvard School of Public Health involved nearly 4,300 teenage boys and found that those who drank more than two servings of skim milk each day had a much higher incidence of acne than those who drank no milk. The research team theorized that skim milk may contain bovine hormones that influence teens' natural growth hormones, which would make young people more susceptible to developing acne.

The 2009 study of Iranian teenagers also found an association between diet and the onset of acne. Even though heredity was determined to be the most significant risk factor, the researchers concluded that "a genetic background can be modified by environmental factors" and "certain nutrition habits may affect acne severity."[44] Specifically, the teenagers who regularly ate sweets, nuts, chocolates, and oily foods suffered from more severe cases of acne than those who did not.

> " In July 2011 researchers from Germany announced a study that may help clear up the mystery of why the T cells in people with psoriasis malfunction the way they do. "

Diets heavy in spicy foods were also evaluated, and the researchers found that these were not associated with acne.

Viral Culprits

A number of skin disorders are the direct result of infection with viruses. Warts, for instance, are noncancerous skin growths caused by the human papillomavirus (HPV). Princeton University Health Services writes: "Each person's immune system deals with HPV differently, so not everyone will develop warts. The incubation period is typically about 3 months, but warts may lie dormant for years. Once HPV has entered your body, whether you develop warts or not, the virus will live in your system forever."[45] The two most common types are common warts and plantar warts. Although common warts may develop anywhere on the body, they usually develop on the fingers or backs of the hands. Plantar warts are deeper, often grow in clusters, and are usually found on the soles of the feet.

> **Genital warts, which are spread through sexual contact with an infected person, are also caused by HPV infection but not by the same types that cause common warts.**

Genital warts, which are spread through sexual contact with an infected person, are also caused by HPV infection but not by the same types that cause common warts. Scientists have identified over 100 HPV subtypes, of which about 10 have been connected with genital warts. According to the AAD, at least half of people who have had sex have been infected with HPV, but many never know it because their immune systems fight the virus off. The group writes: "People who have a weakened immune system may not be able to fight the virus. When the body cannot fight HPV, genital warts can grow."[46]

Another virus connected with skin disorders is the herpes simplex virus, of which there are two types: HSV-1 and HSV-2. The most common symptoms of infection with HSV-1 are clusters of tiny blisters near the mouth or cold sores on the lips. The virus is highly contagious and spreads easily through kissing, touching an infected person's skin, or sharing objects such as tableware or lip balm. HSV-2 is the usual cause of genital herpes, which is spread through sexual contact. Symptoms of genital herpes include pain and/or itching, accompanied by bumps and blisters in the genital area.

Once a person is infected with the herpes virus, it stays in the bloodstream. Symptoms might appear shortly after infection, or the virus might remain dormant until a trigger, such as a fever, menstruation, or emotional stress, causes symptoms to develop. As is the case with HPV, most people who have been infected with the herpes virus never know it; as the Mayo Clinic writes: "The signs and symptoms of HSV can be so mild that they go unnoticed."[47]

More Questions than Answers

Medical researchers are relatively certain about the cause of some skin disorders. For example, numerous studies have shown a connection between UV radiation and skin cancer, whereas acne and psoriasis are more puzzling. Research has shown that heredity plays a major role in the development of these disorders, but not everyone who is genetically predisposed develops them. Thus, certain environmental triggers must also be involved. Infections by viruses like HPV and herpes simplex cause eruptions on the skin in various parts of the body, but with these, also, many people never develop symptoms. In the future, scientists will undoubtedly learn more about the causes of these and other skin disorders, which will lead to the development of better ways to treat and prevent them.

What Causes Acne and Skin Disorders?

> "There is now good evidence that acne can be related to diet."

—CDC Clinics, "Acne/Scarring," 2011. www.cdc-clinics.com.

CDC Clinics is a skin care treatment center in Victoria, Australia.

> "No evidence exists on the role of diet in acne."

—Apostolos Pappas, "The Relationship of Diet and Acne," *Dermatoendocrinol*, September/October 2009. www.ncbi.nlm.nih.gov.

Pappas is a biochemist with the Johnson & Johnson Skin Research Center.

> "Historically, the relationship between diet and acne has been highly controversial."

—Whitney P. Bowe, Smita S. Joshi, and Alan R. Shalita, "Diet and Acne," *Journal of the American Academy of Dermatology*, July 2010. www.ncbi.nlm.nih.gov.

Bowe, Joshi, and Shalita are with the Department of Dermatology at the State University of New York Downstate Medical Center.

Bracketed quotes indicate conflicting positions.

* Editor's Note: While the definition of a primary source can be narrowly or broadly defined, for the purposes of Compact Research, a primary source consists of: 1) results of original research presented by an organization or researcher; 2) eyewitness accounts of events, personal experience, or work experience; 3) first-person editorials offering pundits' opinions; 4) government officials presenting political plans and/or policies; 5) representatives of organizations presenting testimony or policy.

❝Sunlamps and tanning beds promise consumers a bronzed body year-round, but the ultraviolet (UV) radiation from these devices poses serious health risks.❞

—FDA, "Indoor Tanning: The Risks of Ultraviolet Rays," May 2010. www.fda.gov.

The FDA's mission is to protect and promote public health.

❝Rosacea is not caused by alcohol abuse, as people thought in the past. But in people who have rosacea, drinking alcohol may cause symptoms to get worse (flare).❞

—Palo Alto Medical Foundation, "Rosacea," August 12, 2010. www.pamf.org.

The Palo Alto Medical Foundation specializes in medical care, biomedical research, and education.

❝You can get a fungal infection by touching a person who has one. Some kinds of fungi live on damp surfaces, like the floors in public showers or locker rooms. You can easily pick up a fungus there.❞

—American Academy of Family Physicians, "Tinea Infections: Athlete's Foot, Jock Itch and Ringworm," November 2010. http://familydoctor.org.

The American Academy of Family Physicians is a national medical organization that represents over 100,300 family physicians, family medicine residents, and medical students.

❝A number of health conditions, allergies, genetic factors, physical and mental stressors, and irritants can cause dermatitis.❞

—Mayo Clinic, "Dermatitis," December 8, 2009. www.mayoclinic.com.

The Mayo Clinic is a world-renowned medical facility headquartered in Rochester, Minnesota.

66 **Melanoma, the deadliest form of skin cancer, is linked to getting severe sunburns, especially at a young age.** 99

—FDA, "Indoor Tanning: The Risks of Ultraviolet Rays," May 2010. www.fda.gov.

The FDA's mission is to protect and promote public health.

....

66 **Scabies is caused by tiny mites that are not easily seen by the human eye. They burrow into the skin and cause little red bumps and severe itching, particularly at night.** 99

—American Skin Association, "Scabies," 2011. www.americanskin.org.

The American Skin Association is dedicated to defeating melanoma, other skin cancers, and disease.

....

Facts and Illustrations

What Causes Acne and Skin Disorders?

- A study published in August 2010 by a team of Chinese researchers found that **heredity** was the primary factor in the development of adolescent acne, followed by contributing factors such as mental stress, menstrual disorder, frequent insomnia, high-fat diet, being male, anxiety, and sleeping fewer than eight hours per day.

- According to the University of Maryland Medical Center, acne can be triggered by drugs such as **steroids, testosterone, and estrogen**.

- Chicago dermatologist Maria Tsoukas states that the indoor tanning industry has grown five-fold since 1992, and over that same period of time, melanoma rates have increased by **2 percent** in the general population.

- According to the Portuguese Skin Cancer Association, an estimated **10,000** new cases of skin cancer are diagnosed every year in Portugal, and the majority of the cases are caused by overexposure to the sun.

- The National Cancer Institute states that women who use tanning beds more than once a month are **55 percent** more likely to develop malignant melanoma.

- According to the NIH, even though research has shown that chocolate, nuts, and greasy foods do not cause acne, diets high in **refined sugars** may be related to the condition.

Facts and Illustrations

45

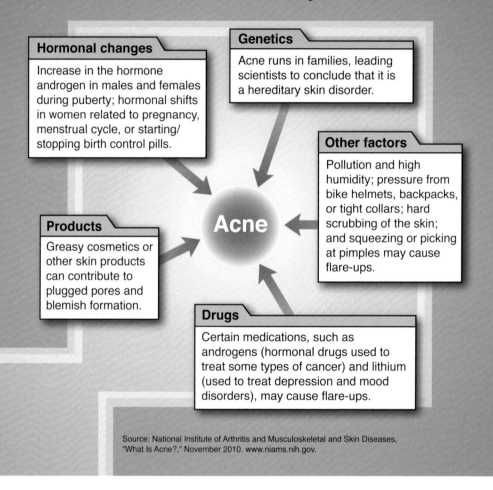

Many Possible Causes of Acne

Scientists are not certain exactly what causes acne. They have identified a number of factors that might contribute to acne, either alone or together.

Hormonal changes
Increase in the hormone androgen in males and females during puberty; hormonal shifts in women related to pregnancy, menstrual cycle, or starting/stopping birth control pills.

Genetics
Acne runs in families, leading scientists to conclude that it is a hereditary skin disorder.

Other factors
Pollution and high humidity; pressure from bike helmets, backpacks, or tight collars; hard scrubbing of the skin; and squeezing or picking at pimples may cause flare-ups.

Products
Greasy cosmetics or other skin products can contribute to plugged pores and blemish formation.

Acne

Drugs
Certain medications, such as androgens (hormonal drugs used to treat some types of cancer) and lithium (used to treat depression and mood disorders), may cause flare-ups.

Source: National Institute of Arthritis and Musculoskeletal and Skin Diseases, "What Is Acne?," November 2010. www.niams.nih.gov.

- The Palo Alto Medical Foundation states that people have a higher risk of developing skin cancer if they live where **UV radiation** is highest, such as areas close to the equator and at higher altitudes.

- The US Environmental Protection Agency states that up to **90 percent** of the visible skin changes commonly attributed to aging are caused by the sun.

Artificial Tanning and Melanoma

For years proponents of indoor tanning claimed that it was safer than natural sunlight, but research has proved that contention to be false. In 2009 the International Agency for Research on Cancer raised artificial tanning devices to its highest cancer risk category of "carcinogenic to humans." A study published in June 2010 found that a large percentage of melanoma patients had used indoor tanning for 10 or more years, and a similarly high percentage had used indoor tanning for 2 to 5 years.

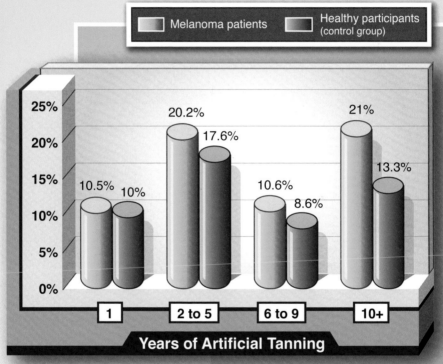

Melanoma patients

Healthy participants (control group)

	1	2 to 5	6 to 9	10+
Melanoma patients	10.5%	20.2%	10.6%	21%
Healthy participants	10%	17.6%	8.6%	13.3%

Years of Artificial Tanning

Source: DeAnn Lazovich et al. "Indoor Tanning and Risk of Melanoma: A Case-Control Study in a Highly Exposed Population," *Cancer Epidemiology, Biomarkers & Prevention*, June 2010. http://cebp.aacrjournals.org.

- According to the Mayo Clinic, the inflammatory skin disease **stasis dermatitis** develops when fluid accumulates in the tissues just beneath the skin (typically the lower legs) due to a sluggish return of blood from the leg veins back to the heart.

Causes of Dermatitis

Dermatitis (also called eczema) is one of the most common skin disorders. Although the cause is unknown, scientists have identified a number of contributing factors. The various types of dermatitis and known triggers are shown.

Type	Symptoms	Possible Causes
Contact dermatitis	Rash, bumps, blisters, itchiness	Genetics, direct contact with irritants (laundry soap, skin soaps/detergents, cleaning products), or allergens (rubber; metals; perfumes; cosmetics; weeds such as poison ivy, oak, or sumac)
Atopic dermatitis	Chronic, itchy rash that comes and goes	Malfunctions of body's immune system; genetic tendency for allergic conditions, such as asthma or hay fever
Neuro-dermatitis	Itchiness in specific areas of skin such as ankles, wrists, outer forearm or arm, and back of neck	Genetics, dry skin, chronic irritation, another type of dermatitis, psoriasis
Seborrheic dermatitis	Red rash with yellowish, somewhat oily scales on the face and scalp (leads to dandruff and known as "cradle cap" in infants)	Genetics, stress, fatigue, neurological conditions such as Parkinson's disease
Stasis dermatitis	Buildup of fluid under the skin of the legs causes swelling and itching	Age (most common among the elderly); varicose veins; other chronic conditions/recurrent infections that affect leg circulation
Perioral dermatitis	Bumpy rash around the mouth (may be a form of the skin disorder rosacea, as symptoms are similar)	Cosmetics, moisturizers, topical cortizone creams, dental products containing fluoride

Source: Mayo Clinic, "Dermatitis," December 8, 2009. www.mayoclinic.com.

- The AAD states that genetic factors and **immune system deficiencies** are involved in the development of melanoma.

- The Skin Cancer Foundation states that 10 minutes in a **tanning bed** matches the cancer-causing effects of 10 minutes in the Mediterranean summer sun.

How Are Acne and Skin Disorders Treated?

❝Benzoyl peroxide and salicylic acid are the most common and most effective over-the-counter medicines for acne. These medicines kill bacteria, dry up the oil and make your skin peel off.❞

—American Academy of Family Physicians, a national medical organization that represents over 100,300 family physicians, family medicine residents, and medical students.

❝Time is of the essence, and when caught early, many forms of skin cancer can be successfully treated.❞

—Robert A. Norman, a dermatologist from Tampa, Florida.

Michael Khalili was 11 years old when he developed vitiligo, a skin pigment disorder that causes white blotches to form on different parts of the body. His first symptoms were small, light-colored patches on his knees, eyelids, and chin, which eventually faded away on their own. During his teens a tiny white patch appeared on his knuckle, but that also went away. Then when Khalili was 23 he says the vitiligo "came back with a vengeance."[48] At first he did not notice the white patches because he has rather pale skin and usually stayed out of the sun. But when he began spending more time in sunny Los Angeles, his skin started to tan and the changes in his appearance were shocking. "This time it didn't go away on its own," he says. "This time I had to actively fight it."[49]

> **Although treatment recommendations vary based on the severity of the outbreak, the overall goal for any acne remedy is to reduce the production of sebum, help the skin shed dead cells so they do not build up, and prevent bacteria from accumulating.**

Khalili visited a dermatologist, who put him on a treatment program that involved sessions of UV light therapy three to four times a week, along with regular application of prescription creams to his skin. But he was careless about sticking to the treatment—and he suffered because of it. In August 2010 he wrote on his blog: "The vitiligo is spreading like wildfire. I'm freaking out. This isn't cool. I don't really mind it on my hands and other parts of my body but my face is seriously starting to look like The Joker [villain in *Batman* movies]." Seeing these skin changes scared Khalili into being more disciplined, as he wrote: "No more . . . excuses. No more flaking on treatment. No more Joker face."[50] This time he was serious about following his doctor's advice, and his newfound resolve paid off. In January 2011 he posted an update on his progress, saying that the white patches were finally starting to fade.

The Right and Wrong Way to Attack Acne

Vitiligo is severely disfiguring and much more challenging to treat than acne. But there was a time when acne was also considered a stubborn skin disorder that was hard to get rid of. Today it can be successfully treated in a variety of ways. Although treatment recommendations vary based on the severity of the outbreak, the overall goal for any acne remedy is to reduce the production of sebum, help the skin shed dead cells so they do not build up, and prevent bacteria from accumulating. According to the NIH, acne medications reduce clumps of cells in the hair follicles and reduce oil production, bacteria, and inflammation.

Dermatologist Jenny Kim first advises her acne patients to wash their skin with a mild cleanser and to use a nonirritating moisturizer that contains sunscreen. Over-the-counter products often contain salicylic acid, which helps prevent clogged pores by slowing the shedding of cells inside the hair follicles, or benzoyl peroxide, which helps remove excess oils from the skin and dead skin cells that clog pores. While both of these ingredients can be beneficial in controlling acne, Kim urges patients to avoid using too many different products at once. She explains: "The old adage 'less is more' applies to patients with sensitive skin. The best advice is to discuss your skin care regimen with your dermatologist who can recommend products based on not only your specific skin condition, but your individual skin type as well."[51]

Sometimes people with acne become so desperate for their skin to clear up that they resort to drastic measures. One teenage girl posted in an online dermatology forum that she had reached the point of being willing to try anything to get rid of her acne. So when she read in a magazine about using nail polish remover as a facial toner, she decided to try it—and she soon learned what a terrible mistake that was. "What they didn't specify was the amount to use," she says. "I stupidly bathed my entire face in it, giving myself quite a severe chemical burn—which lasted a good 3 months and was freshly humiliating every time I had to explain to horrified people that I had done it to myself in pursuit of clear skin."[52]

> " Even after the acne itself has been successfully treated, the skin can remain scarred and pitted from the tissue damage caused by lesions. "

Lingering Scars

One of the most frustrating and painful aspects of acne for many sufferers is the physical scars it leaves behind. Even after the acne itself has been successfully treated, the skin can remain scarred and pitted from the tissue damage caused by lesions. Acne scars can be challenging to treat, but there is hope for those who are troubled by them. For mild scarring, dermatologists may recommend chemical peels, laser treatments, or a process known as microdermabrasion, which is often referred to as a "power peel." This technique, according to a February 2011 article on WebMD, "is more like softened sandblasting."[53] The dermatologist holds a device that sprays tiny crystals while circulating in a gentle abrasion technique that resurfaces the skin by removing its dead outer layer. For some people the treatment may need to be repeated several times in order to achieve the desired result.

A technique used for more serious, deeper acne scars is known as fractional laser resurfacing. The purpose of this treatment is to damage tiny columns of scarred skin by heat-treating them, while leaving surrounding healthy skin intact. Kim explains: "One of the main benefits of fractional resurfacing is wound healing and increased collagen production that reduces acne scars. However, most patients will notice only a modest improvement in acne scarring and multiple treatments are required."[54] Kim adds that to treat the worst acne scars, several different surgical procedures can be used. One is known as punch grafting (or punch excision), in which scar tissue is removed, raised, and/or separated from the underlying skin. Says Kim, "These surgical procedures in combination with other therapies, including lasers and fillers, can produce improvement for severe acne scarring."[55]

> **The ultimate goal of skin cancer treatment is for every trace of cancerous tissue to be removed.**

Fighting Skin Cancer

Skin cancer patients have more hope than ever before of being cured. According to the AAD, dermatologists take a number of factors into consideration before recommending a particular treatment method. These include the type of skin cancer (along with the number of tumors), where it appears on the body, whether it is an aggressive form of cancer, what stage it is in (or how deeply it has grown and/or spread), and the patient's overall health.

The ultimate goal of skin cancer treatment is for every trace of cancerous tissue to be removed. One surgical technique, known as Mohs surgery, is performed only by a dermatologist who has completed specialized medical training. The surgeon first removes the visible part of the skin cancer. Then, because cells are too tiny to be seen with the naked eye, he or she also removes some normal-looking skin that may contain cancerous cells. The surgery is performed one layer at a time, as the AAD writes:

> After removing a layer of skin, it is prepared so that the surgeon can examine it under a microscope and look for cancer cells. If the surgeon sees cancer cells, the surgeon removes another layer of skin. This layer-by-layer approach continues until the surgeon no longer finds cancer cells. In most cases, Mohs surgery can be completed within a day or less. The cure rate for skin cancer is high when Mohs surgery is used.[56]

Melissa DeLuca Nowicki, who is an esthetician (skin care specialist), underwent Mohs surgery in December 2010. She had noticed a small pinkish-colored spot on her forehead and assumed that it was just a dry patch of skin. But rather than going away, it grew and then began to bleed, so Nowicki went to a dermatologist, who performed a biopsy. "Much to my surprise," she writes, "the results came back as a 'basal cell carcinoma.'"[57] The spot was excised from Nowicki's forehead, after which the doctor performed Mohs surgery so that all cancerous cells could be removed.

Freezing-Cold Treatment

A number of skin growths can be removed through a process known as cryotherapy (or cryosurgery), which involves using liquid nitrogen to freeze the lesions off. This technique is common in treating warts, especially plantar warts because they are rooted deep in the skin. The Mayo Clinic writes: "Your doctor can apply liquid nitrogen with a spray canister or cotton-tipped applicator to freeze and destroy your wart. The chemical causes a blister to form around your wart, and the dead tissue sloughs off within a week or so. The application itself can be painful, and cryotherapy can result in painful or tender blisters that resolve on their own."[58]

Another skin condition that is commonly treated with cryotherapy is actinic keratosis, which is a precancerous growth. These growths commonly form on areas of the skin that have had the most sun exposure, and if not removed they can become cancerous. This was shown in a 2009 study that focused on the progression of actinic keratoses to nonmelanoma skin cancers. The researchers found that nearly 65 percent of squamous cell carcinomas and 36 percent of primary basal cell carcinomas arose from clinically diagnosed actinic keratoses. Studies have shown that cryotherapy is extremely effective in treating actinic keratosis, with cure rates ranging from 75 to 99 percent.

A Melanoma Miracle?

Since Dr. Keith Flaherty performed his medical residency in the 1990s, he has been passionate about helping patients who suffer from cancer. A foe of chemotherapy because it destroys healthy cells as well as cancerous cells, Flaherty became fascinated with what he calls the "targeted therapy revolution," meaning the development of drugs designed to target and fix genetic mutations that cause cancer. Targeted therapy, he says, has immense potential "because it is based on what makes cancer tick."[59] For years Flaherty's particular interest has been melanoma, as the deadly skin cancer kills the vast majority of patients whose disease progresses to advanced stages.

> " A number of skin growths can be removed through a process known as cryotherapy (or cryosurgery), which involves using liquid nitrogen to freeze the lesions off. "

In 2008 Flaherty set up an experimental human trial with a drug known as PLX4032. It had been tested in mice that were bred to have a genetic mutation called B-RAF, which is found in many patients with melanoma. When given the drug, the creatures' tumors stopped growing and there were no side effects. Fueled by his excitement over what this might mean for melanoma sufferers, Flaherty recruited a group of advanced-stage melanoma patients who had the same genetic mutation. He warned them that he could not guarantee the outcome, and also that there were risks involved with taking a drug that had never been given to humans. But his cautionary words had no effect on their eagerness to participate, as they all knew this was their last hope.

Just a few weeks after the trial began, most participants started seeing marked improvement. Elmer Bucksbaum had cancerous tumors on his neck, liver, and lungs, and one month after taking the experimental drug his tumors were gone. Mark Bunting, whose melanoma had spread into his bones, was cancer-free after two months in the trial. Christopher Nelson was so desperately ill that he could no longer walk or eat, and his family had been advised to bring in hospice to make him comfortable during his last days of life. After Nelson started taking PLX4032 his progress astounded Flaherty, who remarked that he had never seen a melanoma patient who was so sick improve in such a dramatic way.

As miraculous as these patients' improvement was, however, the drug could not cure them. Their cancer eventually spread and all of them died—but their involvement in the trial bought them precious time that they would not have had otherwise. Bucksbaum and Nelson, for instance, survived nearly a year after taking their first dose of the drug, while Bunting lived for almost three years. Their deaths were heartbreaking for Flaherty, but the amazing progress they made strengthens his confidence in the future of targeted drug therapy for cancer sufferers. He is convinced that the answer lies in combining PLX4032 with other targeted therapy drugs that can collectively stop additional genetic mutations from forming. "We just need to find the right combination," Flaherty says.[60]

Optimism and Hope

Just as no two skin disorders are exactly the same, treatments differ widely. Acne can often be brought under control through a combination of diligent cleansing and topical solutions, and scars can be removed by a variety of surgical techniques. Cryotherapy can get rid of warts as well as precancerous growths, and early treatment can remove most skin cancers. In the future, treatments will likely be improved and expanded, which means that fewer people will have to suffer from the effects of skin disorders.

How Are Acne and Skin Disorders Treated?

—Rebecca Penzer and Steven Ersser, *Principles of Skin Care*. West Sussex, England: Wiley, 2010.

Penzer is a dermatology nurse specialist and Ersser is chair in Nursing Development and Skin Care Research at Bournemouth University in the United Kingdom.

"Treatment is possible, and the good news is, the extremely effective and inexpensive treatment makes it possible for all acne sufferers to get their much desired relief. No one ever has to put up with acne!**"**

—Melanie Vasseur, *Under My Skin*. Campbell, CA: FastPencil, 2010.

Vasseur is a nutritional cosmetic chemist and medical esthetician from San Diego, California.

* Editor's Note: While the definition of a primary source can be narrowly or broadly defined, for the purposes of Compact Research, a primary source consists of: 1) results of original research presented by an organization or researcher; 2) eyewitness accounts of events, personal experience, or work experience; 3) first-person editorials offering pundits' opinions; 4) government officials presenting political plans and/or policies; 5) representatives of organizations presenting testimony or policy.

Primary Source Quotes

66 The vast majority of squamous cell carcinomas are curable when identified and removed in a timely manner. 99

—Skin Cancer Foundation, "Treating Squamous Cell Carcinoma with Mohs Surgery," 2011. www.skincancer.org.

The Skin Cancer Foundation is dedicated to reducing the incidence of skin cancer through research, public education, and awareness.

66 Thanks to advances in medicine, today, virtually every case of acne can be controlled. 99

—AAD, "What Causes Acne?," April 14, 2010. www.aad.org.

Composed of over 17,000 dermatologists, the AAD is dedicated to education, research, and patient advocacy.

66 Topical steroids have been the standard treatment for eczema, with oral steroids being prescribed only for severe flare-ups. 99

—National Eczema Association, "Eczema Quick Fact Sheet," July 10, 2011. www.nationaleczema.org.

Through research, support, and education, the National Eczema Association seeks to improve the health and quality of life for people with eczema.

66 If you are using steroids to get rid of these skin conditions—and many doctors are—you are not curing, you are just suppressing temporarily. 99

—Julia Tatum Hunter, interviewed by Roby Mitchell, "Treating Skin Disorders from the Inside Out: An Interview with Dr. Julia Hunter," *Holistic Primary Care*, Winter 2010. www.holisticprimarycare.net.

Hunter is a holistic dermatologist from Beverly Hills, California.

❝Doctors can prescribe medicines and other treatments for rosacea. There is no cure, but with treatment, most people can control their symptoms and keep the disease from getting worse.❞

—Palo Alto Medical Foundation, "Rosacea," August 12, 2010. www.pamf.org.

The Palo Alto Medical Foundation specializes in medical care, biomedical research, and education.

❝A number of natural options have been studied as possible treatments for dermatitis. Although none are as potent as steroid medications, natural approaches generally aren't associated with the same risk of side effects.❞

—Mayo Clinic, "Dermatitis: Alternative Medicine," December 8, 2009. www.mayoclinic.com.

The Mayo Clinic is a world-renowned medical facility headquartered in Rochester, Minnesota.

❝Researchers continue to work on developing new drugs to treat acne. They're also trying to better understand the causes of acne so they can explore new remedies.❞

—NIH, "Understanding Acne," *NIH News in Health*, January 2010. http://newsinhealth.nih.gov.

The NIH is the United States' leading medical research agency.

❝Melanoma is almost always curable when it is detected in its early stages.❞

—American Cancer Society, "Skin Cancer Facts," April 30, 2010. www.cancer.org.

The American Cancer Society seeks to eliminate cancer through research, education, advocacy, and service.

How Are Acne and
Skin Disorders Treated?

- According to dermatologist Robert A. Norman, treating **acne** at an early stage helps lessen the severity of damage to tissue, which prevents or decreases scarring.

- Melanie Vasseur, who is a nutritional cosmetic chemist and medical esthetician from San Diego, California, says that only **11 percent** of people who suffer from acne seek medical attention from a doctor.

- According to internal medicine physicians Christine Laine and David R. Goldmann, moderate to severe acne often requires both topical (applied directly to the skin) and oral **(antibiotics and hormonal agents)** treatments.

- The Skin Cancer Foundation states that the average survival rate for people whose melanoma is detected and treated before it spreads is **99 percent.**

- According to the AAD, **birth control pills** that contain the hormones estrogen and progestin help control acne in women.

- Dermatologist Julia Tatum Hunter states that severe acne and many other skin disorders can improve or disappear when **gut (intestinal) inflammation** is detected and treated.

Promising Developments in Skin Disorder Treatment

A June 2011 report by the Pharmaceutical Research and Manufacturers of America revealed that nearly 300 medicines to treat skin disorders are currently in development. In a sampling of medicines being developed for skin disorders (shown below), the largest number are devoted to the treatment of skin cancer and skin infections.

Number of medicines being developed for skin disorders:

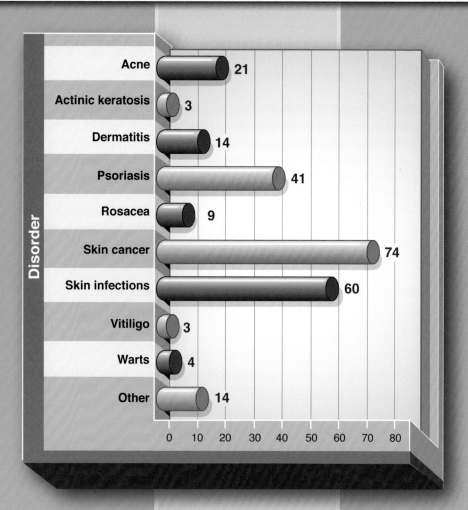

Source: Pharmaceutical Research and Manufacturers of America, "Biopharmaceutical Research Companies Are Developing 300 Medicines to Treat Diseases of the Skin," *Medicines in Development for Skin Disease*, June 2011. www.phrma.org.

Surgical Skin Cancer Treatments

Health officials say that all types of skin cancer are nearly 100 percent curable if they are caught early enough. Before choosing which treatment to use, a dermatologist takes into consideration such factors as the type of skin cancer, where it appears on the body, whether it is aggressive, the stage (how deeply the skin cancer has grown and whether it has spread), and the patient's health. If the cancer has not spread, the dermatologist often surgically removes it. This table shows some of the surgical treatments for skin cancer.

Treatment	Procedure
Excision	The dermatologist numbs the skin and surgically cuts out the growth, along with a small amount of normal-looking skin (called a margin) to ensure complete removal of the cancer.
Curettage and electrodesiccation (used for small basal cell and squamous cell skin cancers)	The dermatologist scrapes the growth with a long, spoon-shaped instrument called a curette, and then uses an electric needle to gently cauterize (burn) the remaining cancer cells, as well as a small amount of normal-looking tissue. The scraping and cauterizing process is usually repeated three times, and the wound tends to heal without stitches.
Mohs surgery (performed only by a dermatologist who has received specialized medical training)	This type of surgery is performed one layer at a time. The Mohs surgeon removes the visible part of the skin cancer, along with some normal-looking skin that may contain cancer cells, and examines the tissue under a microscope. If any cancer cells can be seen, another layer of skin is removed, and this layer-by-layer technique is repeated until no cancer cells are visible.

Source: American Academy of Dermatology, "Skin Cancer: Diagnosis, Treatment, and Outcome," 2011. www.aad.org.

- According to New Jersey physician Manny Alvarez, risks associated with the acne treatment **Accutane** include kidney failure, heart problems, and death.

- According to a November 2010 article on the health information website WebMD, even people with severe psoriasis can get relief during flare-ups in about **85 to 95 percent** of cases.

- Princeton University Health Services states that **warts** can be treated or removed, but most disappear on their own in two years.

- According to the health insurance provider Cigna, **one out of four** people who develop the bacterial infection called necrotizing fasciitis (flesh-eating disease) die from it.

- The Skin Cancer Foundation states that the overall melanoma survival rate for African Americans is **77 percent**, compared with **91 percent** for Caucasians.

- The AAD cautions that some natural supplements used to treat acne have been found to contain over **200** times the amount of the mineral selenium stated on the label, which can lead to selenium poisoning.

- According to internal medicine physicians Christine Laine and David R. Goldmann, some experts believe that **acne surgery** produces a rapid improvement in appearance, but no scientific evidence has confirmed that this is superior to drug therapy alone.

Can Acne and Skin Disorders Be Prevented?

> **The pimply millions rely on infomercial products hawked by celebrities or over-the-counter lotions, cleansers, and topical remedies. Recent research suggests that it's not what we slather on our skin that matters most but what we put in our mouth.**

—Mark Hyman, who is a physician and the founder of Acne Wellness Center in Lenox, Massachusetts.

> **The best ways to lower the risk of non-melanoma skin cancer are to avoid intense sunlight for long periods of time and to practice sun safety. You can continue to exercise and enjoy the outdoors while practicing sun safety at the same time.**

—American Cancer Society, which seeks to eliminate cancer through research, education, advocacy, and service.

After Joel Myres died of melanoma, some of his fellow medical students at the University of California at Irvine wanted to do something to honor his memory. Myres had battled the disease since he was 16 years old. His friends theorized that, like him, sun-loving teenagers were likely unaware of the risks posed by skin cancer. As a way of addressing the lack of awareness, the students developed an educational program targeted at teens in grades 6 to 12. The authors of an April 2010 paper about the program explain: "Because sun exposure during youth appears particularly important to melanoma risk, and because habits and attitudes pertaining to sun protection behavior are presumably formed early in life, it is crucial to teach our youth the importance of sun safety and skin cancer awareness."[61] The program educates teenagers about skin structure and function, the three main types of skin cancer, and effects of UV radiation. Also covered is the importance of self-screening for early detection, which is emphasized with the message "Spot a spot, save a life!"[62]

> "The AAD, NIH, and other related health organizations say that most cases of skin cancer can be prevented.

The success of the program has been phenomenal. What began as a local effort that involved a few medical student volunteers and just over 1,000 teenagers has grown into the National Melanoma Awareness Project, with over 25 medical school chapters educating thousands of teens each year. The April 2010 paper sums up the value of programs such as this one in helping young people to be aware of the dangers of skin cancer and to know how to prevent it: "Medical students can act as a tremendous asset to health awareness public outreach efforts: enthusiastic volunteerism keeps education cost-effective, results in exponential spread of information, reinforces knowledge and communication skills of future physicians, and can result in tangible, life-saving benefits such as early detection of melanoma."[63]

Stopping Skin Cancer Before It Starts

The AAD, NIH, and other related health organizations say that most cases of skin cancer can be prevented. Because of the strong link between the disease and UV radiation, recommended preventive measures always emphasize the importance of protection from the sun. One of the primary warnings is for people to avoid being in the sun during the middle of the day, and that is true no matter what time of year it is. The Mayo Clinic writes: "For many people in North America, the sun's rays are strongest between about 10 a.m. and 4 p.m. Schedule outdoor activities for other times of the day, even in winter or when the sky is cloudy. You absorb UV radiation year-round, and clouds offer little protection from damaging rays."[64]

With the rapid proliferation of tanning salons throughout the United States, health officials are becoming more aggressive in their warnings about the dangers of artificial tanning. Studies continue to show that UV radiation from tanning devices can play as much of a role in the development of skin cancer as the UV rays from natural sunlight—yet the AAD says that an estimated 28 million people in the United States, including over 2 million teenagers, tan indoors each year. Since avoiding these devices can go a long way toward helping prevent skin cancer, the AAD supports a ban on the production and sale of indoor tanning equipment for nonmedical purposes. In lieu of such a ban, the group supports restrictions that prohibit indoor tanning facilities from using advertisements with verbiage such as "safe," "safe tanning," "no harmful rays," "no adverse effect," or any similar wording.

Another crucial element in preventing skin cancer is regular examination of the body to check for abnormal moles, suspicious spots, or growths. The face, neck, ears, and scalp should be checked regularly, as should the chest and trunk, both fronts and backs of legs, and the feet, including the soles and spaces between toes. Melissa DeLuca Nowicki is someone who understands the importance of early detection. After Nowicki had a basal cell carcinoma removed from her forehead in December 2010, she began to wonder about a spot on her shoulder and asked the dermatologist to biopsy it. "At the worst," she says, "we thought maybe it would be another basal cell carcinoma, well boy were we wrong."[65] The biopsy revealed that the spot was an abnormal lesion that contained melanoma cells. As it turned out, though, early detection had kept the cancer in check and may have saved Nowicki's life. She writes:

> **Dermatologists and health organizations widely agree that using sunscreen is an essential preventive measure for all types of skin cancer.**

> The biopsy was not titled "melanoma" because it was in the early stages, but the urgency to have it removed was the

same. A day later the doctor did a wide-margin excision on my right shoulder to attempt to completely remove the lesion. Two weeks later, results were in and my shoulder was completely clear! That was great news, due to early detection, a baby melanoma was stopped in its tracks.[66]

The Skinny on Sunscreen

Dermatologists and health organizations widely agree that using sunscreen is an essential preventive measure for all types of skin cancer. But because consumers can easily get confused about which sunscreens are the most effective (and which barely protect at all), the FDA developed stringent testing and labeling criteria for product manufacturers, which was announced in June 2011. One requirement applies to use of the term *broad spectrum*, which indicates that a sunscreen protects against UVA and UVB rays, both of which can cause skin cancer. In order for the term to be used, manufacturers must submit their products for FDA testing to prove that their sunscreens provide this broad protection.

The new FDA rules also apply to sun protection factor (SPF) values, which measure a sunscreen's effectiveness against UV rays. Higher numbers indicate greater protection, as the Skin Cancer Foundation explains: "For instance, someone using a sunscreen with an SPF of 15 will take 15 times longer to redden than without the sunscreen. An SPF 15 sunscreen screens 93 percent of the sun's UVB rays; SPF 30 protects against 97 percent; and SPF 50, 98 percent."[67] Under the new requirements, only sunscreens with SPF of 15 or higher may state on labels that they reduce the risk of skin cancer and premature aging of the skin. Moreover, any sunscreens that do not fit the criteria for broad spectrum, or that are broad spectrum but have SPF values between 2 to 14, are required to have warning labels clearly stating that the product cannot help prevent skin cancer or early skin aging.

The FDA has also proposed regulatory criteria that would allow it to

> **Steps can be taken that help keep people from developing the rashes and blisters that are the hallmark of dermatitis.**

limit the maximum SPF value shown on sunscreen labels. According to the FDA, this is necessary because research has not shown that products with SPF values higher than 50 provide greater protection than those with SPF values of 50. Without such guidelines, consumers could buy sunscreen labeled SPF 100 and be unaware that they are getting no more protection than they would with SPF 50.

Heading Off Dermatitis

Scientists know that people who develop dermatitis suffer from some sort of overactive inflammatory response to irritating substances, which causes their skin to itch. Beyond that, however, much remains unknown—meaning that dermatitis cannot be prevented. But steps can be taken that help keep people from developing the rashes and blisters that are the hallmark of dermatitis. For instance, those who are sensitive to the sap urushiol need to become very familiar with plants such as poison ivy, oak, and sumac and must go out of their way to avoid contact with them. Preventive measures can also be taken to avoid outbreaks of other types of dermatitis, as the Mayo Clinic explains: "Try to identify and avoid triggers that worsen the inflammation. Rapid changes of temperature, sweating and stress can worsen some forms of dermatitis. Avoid direct contact with wool products, such as rugs, bedding and clothes, as well as harsh soaps and detergents. If you must handle products that irritate your skin, wear nonlatex gloves."[68]

Because dermatitis is often exacerbated by skin that is too dry, sufferers may be able to avoid outbreaks by taking steps to keep their skin from drying out. The Mayo Clinic recommends less frequent bathing, as the group explains: "Most people who are prone to dermatitis don't need to bathe daily. Try going a day or two without a shower or bath. When you do bathe, limit yourself to 15 to 20 minutes, and use warm, rather than hot, water."[69] Other prevention measures include using mild soaps when bathing, patting the skin dry rather than rubbing it, and liberal use of moisturizers that are made for sensitive skin.

Keeping Acne at Bay

As with any disease or disorder for which the exact cause is unknown, acne is not considered to be preventable. If acne runs in someone's family, for instance, genetic factors are involved and little (or nothing) can be done to stop the disorder. The same is true of hormonal changes, which are unavoidable during adolescence and play a significant role in the development of acne. What people can do, however, is take precautions to avoid the environmental triggers that can contribute to breakouts. Keeping the skin clean without excessive washing or scrubbing is an important preventive measure, as is avoiding greasy cosmetics or lotions, oily hair products, or acne concealers, all of which can clog the pores and contribute to acne.

> " As with any disease or disorder for which the exact cause is unknown, acne is not considered to be preventable. "

Also, says the Mayo Clinic, watching what touches one's face can help prevent breakouts: "Keep your hair clean and off your face. Also avoid resting your hands or objects, such as telephone receivers, on your face. Tight clothing or hats also can pose a problem, especially if you'll be sweating. Sweat, dirt and oils can contribute to acne."[70] The group adds that other important acne prevention measures include removing makeup before going to bed, cleaning cosmetic brushes and applicators regularly with soapy water, and showering after exercising or doing strenuous work, as oil and sweat on the skin can trap dirt and bacteria.

Precautions for People of Color

According to the AAD, people who use pomade oil or ointment to style or manage their hair have a high likelihood of developing acne. The AAD says one study of African American acne patients revealed that nearly half used pomade, and over 70 percent of those developed acne on the forehead. The group writes:

> The acne that develops from using pomade is called "acne cosmetica" or "pomade acne." It occurs when pomade blocks pores and acne develops on the scalp, forehead and/or temples—places where pomade comes into contact with the skin. Pomade acne usually consists of blackheads and whiteheads, with perhaps a few papules [small red bumps] and pustules [bumps resembling whiteheads rimmed in red].[71]

In order to avoid developing acne, the AAD recommends that pomade use be limited to areas behind the hairline and on the ends of the hair to keep the product away from the forehead and scalp.

Another skin problem that has been closely connected with pomade use is folliculitis. This is a bacterial infection of the scalp, in which pus-filled bumps and redness develop around the hairline. The disorder can be serious, potentially leading to hair loss and the spread of infection. Since folliculitis is often difficult to treat, the AAD recommends that people take every possible precaution to help prevent it from developing, including discontinuing the use of pomades.

Control and Prevention

Whether skin disorders are preventable is directly related to their cause—if the cause is unknown, or is related to genetics (as many are), there is no way to prevent the disorders. Acne, for instance, is not considered a preventable disorder, but steps can be taken to keep it under control and, in some cases, to avoid breakouts. The same is true with rosacea and psoriasis; neither is preventable, but sufferers can learn to avoid certain triggers that cause flare-ups. Skin cancer is one disease that *can* often be prevented if people heed the advice of health officials and avoid overexposure to UV radiation. As research continues in the future, scientists will undoubtedly clear up many of the mysteries related to skin disorders, meaning that more of them may become preventable.

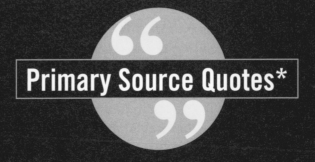

Primary Source Quotes*

Can Acne and Skin Disorders Be Prevented?

66 Sunscreens do not protect against inflammation or UV-induced DNA damage, they simply delay the response. 99

—Julia Tatum Hunter, interviewed by Roby Mitchell, "Treating Skin Disorders from the Inside Out: An Interview with Dr. Julia Hunter," *Holistic Primary Care*, Winter 2010. www.holisticprimarycare.net.

Hunter is a holistic dermatologist from Beverly Hills, California.

66 The American Academy of Dermatology . . . today reiterated the safety and effectiveness of sunscreens to protect against the damaging effects from exposure to ultraviolet (UV) radiation. 99

—AAD, "Sunscreens Remain Safe, Effective Form of Sun Protection," May 23, 2011. www.aad.org.

Composed of over 17,000 dermatologists, the AAD is dedicated to education, research, and patient advocacy.

Bracketed quotes indicate conflicting positions.

* Editor's Note: While the definition of a primary source can be narrowly or broadly defined, for the purposes of Compact Research, a primary source consists of: 1) results of original research presented by an organization or researcher; 2) eyewitness accounts of events, personal experience, or work experience; 3) first-person editorials offering pundits' opinions; 4) government officials presenting political plans and/or policies; 5) representatives of organizations presenting testimony or policy.

"Because hereditary factors seem to play a large role in the development of acne, most primary prevention strategies have not been shown to be effective."

—Christine Laine and David R. Goldmann, *In the Clinic: Practical Information About Common Health Problems.* Philadelphia, PA: ACP, 2009.

Laine and Goldmann are internal medicine physicians from Philadelphia, Pennsylvania.

"While there is no real established link between diet and psoriasis, since psoriasis is connected to heart disease and diabetes . . . , I tell patients to eat a good, balanced diet that's good for your heart, rich in fish oils, for example."

—Paul Yamauchi, interviewed by *Skincare News*, "Psoriasis Expert Dr. Paul Yamauchi Talks About Treating Chronic Skin Conditions," SkinCare-News.com, April 19, 2010. www.skincare-news.com.

Yamauchi is a dermatologist and the medical director of the Dermatology Institute & Skin Care Center of Santa Monica, California.

"Let's face it, sun is no good for your skin. Sunscreens, hats with wide brims, and long sleeves will lower the risk of skin cancer and keep your skin younger looking."

—James M. Fries and Donald M. Vickery, *Take Care of Yourself.* Cambridge, MA: Da Capo, 2009.

Fries is a professor of medicine at Stanford University, and Vickery was head of the nonprofit Self-Care Institute before his death in 2008.

"Azelaic acid (trade name Azelex) is a natural acid found in whole-grain cereals and animal products. This topical cream is thought to help the skin renew itself more quickly and prevent the buildup of cells that can plug pores, thereby reducing pimple and blackhead formation. It also helps to kill . . . the bacteria that causes acne."

—Hope Ricciotti and Monique Doyle Spencer, *The Real Life Body Book.* New York: Random House, 2010.

Ricciotti is an associate professor at Harvard Medical School, and Spencer is an author.

66 Everyone knows about obvious culprits like poison ivy, poison oak and stinging nettles, but for people with eczema trying to avoid any plants with fuzzy leaves and stems is a good idea.99

—National Eczema Association, "Eczema Quick Fact Sheet," July 10, 2011. www.nationaleczema.org.

Through research, support, and education, the National Eczema Association seeks to improve the health and quality of life for people with eczema.

66 Preventing contact dermatitis means avoiding coming into contact with those substances, such as poison ivy or harsh soaps, that may cause it.99

—Mayo Clinic, "Dermatitis: Prevention," December 8, 2009. www.mayoclinic.com.

The Mayo Clinic is a world-renowned medical facility headquartered in Rochester, Minnesota.

66 Childhood exposure to UV and the number of times a child is burnt by UV, either from the sun or from sunbeds, are known to increase the risk of developing melanoma later in life. For this reason, particular attention is required to ensure children and adolescents do not use sunbeds.99

—World Health Organization, "Sunbeds, Tanning and UV Exposure," April 2010. www.who.int.

The World Health Organization is the directing and coordinating authority for health within the United Nations system.

Facts and Illustrations

Can Acne and Skin Disorders Be Prevented?

- According to the FDA, there is no known way to **prevent acne**.

- The Environmental Protection Agency states that unprotected exposure to **UV radiation** (from the sun or tanning beds) is the most preventable risk factor for skin cancer.

- According to the Mayo Clinic, sunscreens do not filter out all harmful UV radiation, especially the **radiation** that can lead to melanoma.

- An October 2010 article on the health information website WebMD states that measures to help prevent **rosacea** include avoiding sun exposure, alcohol, hot foods, spicy foods, intense exercise, and stress.

- According to the children's health system Nemours, the fungal skin infection known as **jock itch** can be prevented by keeping the groin area clean and dry, especially after showering, swimming, and sweaty activities.

- The International Agency for Research on Cancer recommends that commercial **indoor tanning be banned** for those who are under the age of 18 to help prevent skin cancer.

Young Females Ignore Risks of Artificial Tanning

Studies have shown that most skin cancer is preventable if people avoid over-exposure to ultraviolet (UV) rays from the sun and artificial tanning devices. Yet a 2011 survey by the American Academy of Dermatology found that many teen girls and young women are willing to ignore the risks in pursuit of what they perceive as an attractively bronzed body. This graph shows how frequent indoor tanners responded to questions about the risks versus the benefits.

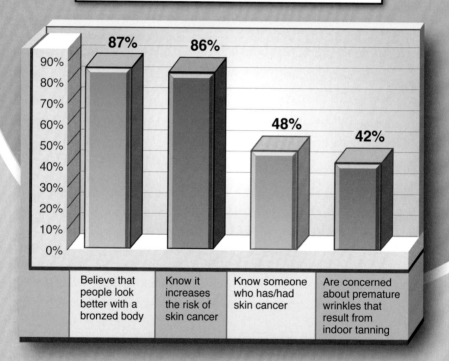

Of girls and young women aged 14 to 22 who used a tanning bed in the past year:

Believe that people look better with a bronzed body	Know it increases the risk of skin cancer	Know someone who has/had skin cancer	Are concerned about premature wrinkles that result from indoor tanning
87%	86%	48%	42%

Source: Marissa Cevallos, "Many Teens Who Tan Know the Cancer Risk but Do It Anyway, Survey Finds," *Los Angeles Times*, May 18, 2011. www.latimes.com.

- According to the Centers for Disease Control and Prevention, a vaccination called **Zostavax** can prevent people from developing a painful, herpes-related skin condition known as **shingles** but will not prevent against other forms of herpes, such as genital herpes.

Healthy Skin Helps Avoid Skin Disorders

Although skin disorders such as acne, psoriasis, rosacea, and dermatitis are not considered to be preventable, taking steps to protect and nurture the skin can often help avoid flare-ups of these disorders.

Mayo Clinic recommendations for keeping skin healthy:

Skin Health tactic	Why Important
Sun protection: Avoid the sun from 10 a.m. to 4 p.m.; apply sunscreen liberally and often; wear protective clothing when in the sun	Helps prevent premature aging, wrinkles, age spots, and more serious problems, such as skin cancer
Avoid smoking	Prevents premature aging of skin; depletion of oxygen and nutrients, such as vitamin A, that contribute to skin health; damage to collagen and elastin (that give skin strength and elasticity)
Gentle skin treatment: Limit bath time, use warm rather than hot water, avoid strong soaps, shave carefully, pat dry rather than rubbing, moisturize dry skin with cream or lotion that fits skin type	As tough and protective as skin is, daily cleansing and shaving can be hard on it; rough, harsh skin treatments and scrubbing can cause flare-ups of acne and other skin disorders
Eat a healthy diet: Plenty of fruits, vegetables, whole grains, and lean proteins	Connection between diet and acne is not clear, but research suggests a healthy diet rich in vitamin C and low in fats and carbohydrates may promote younger looking skin
Manage stress: Set reasonable limits, relax more, scale back on commitments, make time for enjoyable activities	Uncontrolled stress makes skin more sensitive and triggers acne breakouts and other skin problems

Source: Mayo Clinic, "Skin Care: 5 Tips for Healthy Skin," November 24, 2009. www.mayoclinic.com.

State Restrictions on Indoor Tanning for Minors

The American Academy of Dermatology and many other health organizations emphasize that avoiding overexposure to ultraviolet (UV) radiation from the sun and artificial tanning devices is considered the single most important step people can take to prevent skin cancer. Because of the risks involved, 19 states either ban the use of tanning facilities for youth under a certain age or require parental accompaniment, as this map shows.

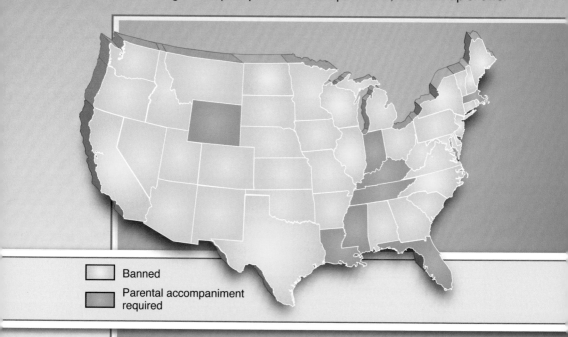

☐ Banned

☐ Parental accompaniment required

Source: National Conference of State Legislatures, "Tanning Restrictions for Minors—A State-by-State Comparison," September 2010. www.ncsl.org.

- Princeton University Health Services states that **foot and toenail fungus** can be prevented by wearing flip-flops or other protective footwear in locker rooms and showers.

- The Palo Alto Medical Foundation states that because **eczema** is hereditary, women can help prevent their babies from developing it by breastfeeding for at least six months in order to boost their immune system.

- According to the Palo Alto Medical Foundation, flare-ups of **psoriasis** may be prevented by avoiding alcohol and smoking, both of which can make the condition worse.

- The children's health system Nemours states that children usually catch the fungal skin infection known as **ringworm** from another infected child; the infection can be prevented by not sharing combs, brushes, pillows, and hats.

- The National Eczema Association states that in addition to avoiding obvious irritants such as **poison ivy**, people with eczema should also avoid citrus fruits, such as lemons, limes, and oranges, and flowers, such as daisies, sunflowers, chrysanthemums, and poinsettias.

Key People and Advocacy Groups

American Academy of Dermatology: The largest and most influential dermatology organization in the United States.

American Cancer Society: An organization that seeks to eliminate cancer and save lives through research, education, advocacy, and service.

American Skin Association: A collaboration of patients, advocates, physicians, and scientists working together to defeat melanoma, other forms of skin cancer, and disease.

Samuel Cooper: A British surgeon who in 1840 was the first to report that melanoma spreads throughout the body and can be treated only through surgical removal of the cancer.

John Hunter: A British physician who first discovered melanoma in 1787 after removing a cancerous tumor from a patient's lower jaw.

Indoor Tanning Association: A trade group that represents indoor tanning equipment manufacturers, distributors, facility owners, and members from other support industries.

Albert Kligman: A dermatologist from Philadelphia, Pennsylvania, who in 1969 found that topical tretinoin (first marketed under the brand name Retin-A) is an effective treatment for acne and also helps repair skin that has been damaged by the sun's UV rays.

René Laennec: A French physician who originated the term *melanoma* and described in an 1804 lecture how the cancer spreads to the lungs.

Henry Oliver Lancaster: An Australian scientist who reported in 1956 that melanoma mortality rates were much higher in areas with more sunlight than in areas with less sunlight.

Skin Cancer Foundation: A group that is dedicated to reducing the incidence of skin cancer through research, public education, and awareness.

Ferdinand Ritter von Hebra: An Austrian dermatologist who was the first to classify skin diseases by structural alterations and to recognize that they are caused by parasites, fungi, and other irritants.

Friedrich Wolff: A German scientist who invented indoor tanning equipment.

Chronology

1906
The German medical company Heraeus introduces the world's first indoor tanning lamp, which is designed to help people suffering from rickets and other skin conditions involving vitamin D deficiency.

1840
British surgeon Samuel Cooper declares that because melanoma spreads throughout the body, a patient's only hope for survival is for the skin cancer to be surgically removed.

1841
Austrian dermatologist Ferdinand Ritter von Hebra coins the term *psoriasis* to describe a skin disease caused by climatic conditions, habits (including consumption of brandy), and nervous temperaments.

1938
Austrian chemist Franz Greiter invents the first sunscreen, called *Gletscher Crème*.

1840   **1900**   **1950**

1857
British physician William Norris publishes a report titled *Eight Cases of Melanosis with Pathological and Therapeutical Remarks on That Disease*, in which he describes a relationship between moles and melanoma.

1896
German dermatologist Paul Gerson Unna publishes the book *The Histopathology of Diseases of the Skin*, in which he reports a link between sun exposure and cancer of the face, neck, and hands.

1943
Para-aminobenzoic acid (PABA) is patented and becomes one of the first UV absorber ingredients to be used in sunscreen; it is later taken off the market after being linked with allergic reactions.

1844
Ferdinand Ritter von Hebra becomes the first to prove that a parasitic itch mite is responsible for a skin disease that later comes to be known as scabies.

2011
The FDA announces its adoption of stringent testing and labeling requirements for manufacturers of sunscreen products.

1962
Franz Greiter introduces the concept of SPF, which becomes the worldwide standard for measuring the effectiveness of sunscreen to shield the sun's harmful UV rays.

2010
A study of more than 1,600 adults in Australia finds that regular use of sunscreen reduces the risk of developing melanoma by at least 50 percent.

2009
The International Agency for Research on Cancer raises artificial tanning devices to its highest cancer risk category of "carcinogenic to humans" from the former rating of "probably carcinogenic to humans."

1984
Albert Kligman reports that tretinoin cream can help repair skin that has been damaged by the sun's UV rays.

1960

1985

2010

1978
Tantrific Sun, the first indoor tanning facility in the United States, opens in Searcy, Arkansas.

2007
A study by researchers from the San Gallicano Dermatological Institute in Rome, Italy, finds that smokers who suffered from acne as teenagers were four times more likely than nonsmokers to develop acne as adults.

1969
Philadelphia dermatologist Albert Kligman reports that tretinoin cream is an effective treatment for acne.

1998
In a presentation to the American Association for the Advancement of Science, scientists from New York's Memorial Sloan-Kettering Cancer Center report that sunscreen protects against sunburn but not melanoma, the deadliest form of skin cancer.

2002
British scientists analyzing hundreds of tumor samples find the same mutated gene, known as B-RAF, in more than half of melanomas.

Related Organizations

American Academy of Dermatology (AAD)

930 E. Woodfield Rd.
PO Box 4014
Schaumburg, IL 60618-4014
phone: (847) 240-1280; toll-free: (866) 503-7546
fax: (847) 240-1859
website: www.aad.org

With over 17,000 dermatologist members, the AAD is the largest and most influential dermatology organization in the United States. Its website offers news releases, skin health tips, information about skin cancer, and a "Dermatology A to Z" section that provides a wealth of educational material about acne and other disorders of the skin.

American Cancer Society (ACS)

250 Williams St. NW, Suite 600
Atlanta, GA 30303
phone: (404) 320-3333 • fax: (404) 982-3677
website: www.cancer.org

The ACS seeks to eliminate cancer and save lives through research, education, advocacy, and service. Its website offers *Cancer Facts & Figures* booklets, a "Stories of Hope" section, a research section, and a searchable "Learn About Cancer" area that provides detailed information about skin cancer.

American Melanoma Foundation (AMF)

3914 Murphy Canyon Rd., Suite A132
San Diego, CA 92123
phone: (858) 277-4426 • fax: (858) 277-4218
e-mail: sunsmartz@melanomafoundation.org
website: www.melanomafoundation.org

The AMF supports research for new melanoma treatments and educates the public about melanoma through awareness programs. Its website offers information about melanoma prevention, diagnosis and treatment, and clinical trials.

American Skin Association (ASA)

6 E. Forty-Third St., 28th Floor
New York, NY 10017
phone: (212) 889-4858 • fax: (212) 889-4959
e-mail: info@americanskin.org • website: www.americanskin.org

The ASA is a collaboration of patients, advocates, physicians, and scientists working together to defeat melanoma, other forms of skin cancer, and disease. Its website has a "Skin Research Center" section that offers information about sun safety, melanoma, "Skin Issues at a Glance," publications, and additional resources.

Centers for Disease Control and Prevention (CDC)

1600 Clifton Rd.
Atlanta, GA 30333
phone: (800) 232-4636 • fax: (770) 488-4760
website: www.cdc.gov

An agency of the US Department of Health and Human Services, the CDC seeks to promote health and quality of life by controlling disease, injury, and disability. Numerous publications about acne and skin disorders can be accessed through the website's search engine.

Indoor Tanning Association (ITA)

2025 M St. NW, Suite 800
Washington, DC 20036
phone: (888) 377-0477 • fax: (202) 367-2142
website: www.theita.com

The ITA is a trade group that represents indoor tanning equipment manufacturers, distributors, facility owners, and members from other support industries. Its website offers news releases and articles related to artificial tanning.

Melanoma Research Foundation (MRF)

1411 K St. NW, Suite 500
Washington, DC 20005
phone: (202) 347-9675; toll-free: (800) 673-1290 • fax: (202) 347-9678
website: www.melanoma.org

The MRF supports medical research and educates patients and physicians about prevention, diagnosis, and treatment of melanoma. Its website features extensive information about melanoma, as well as news releases, patient stories, and research updates.

National Eczema Association (NEA)

4460 Redwood Hwy., Suite 16D
San Rafael, CA 94903-1953
phone: (415) 499-3474; toll-free: (800) 818-7546 • fax: (415) 472-5345
e-mail: info@nationaleczema.org • website: www.nationaleczema.org

The NEA seeks to improve the health and quality of life for people with eczema through research, support, and education. Its website features news releases, an *E-insights* monthly e-newsletter, and a "Living with Eczema" section with treatment videos and informational publications about eczema.

National Institute of Arthritis and Musculoskeletal and Skin Diseases (NIAMS)

1 AMS Cir.
Bethesda, MD 20892-3675
phone: (301) 495-4484; toll-free: (877) 226-4267 • fax: (301) 718-6366
e-mail: NIAMSinfo@mail.nih.gov • website: www.niams.nih.gov

The NIAMS supports research into the causes, treatment, and prevention of arthritis and musculoskeletal and skin diseases, trains scientists to carry out this research, and provides information on research progress. Its website offers news releases, research updates, and a search engine that produces numerous articles about acne and other skin disorders.

National Psoriasis Foundation (NPF)

6600 SW Ninety-Second Ave., Suite 300
Portland, OR 97223-7195
phone: (503) 244-7404; toll-free: (800) 723-9166 • fax: (503) 245-0626
e-mail: getinfo@psoriasis.org • website: www.psoriasis.org

The NPF is dedicated to finding a cure for psoriasis and psoriatic arthritis through research, advocacy, and education. Its website offers news stories, press releases, advocacy news, and an "I Have Psoriasis" section designed to educate people about the illness and its effects.

National Rosacea Society (NRS)

196 James St.
Barrington, IL 60010
phone: (888) 662-5874
e-mail: rosaceas@aol.com • website: www.rosacea.org

The NRS seeks to raise awareness of rosacea, provide public health information about it, and support medical research. Its website offers educational booklets, archived issues of the *Rosacea Review* newsletter, a link to the agency's blog, and an "Information for Patients" section that offers extensive information about rosacea.

Skin Cancer Foundation (SCF)

149 Madison Ave., Suite 901
New York, NY 10016
phone: (212) 725-5176 • fax: (212) 725-5751
e-mail: info@skincancer.org • website: www.skincancer.org

The SCF is dedicated to reducing the incidence of skin cancer through research, public education, and awareness. Its website offers educational information about the different types of skin cancer, a "Skin Cancer Facts" section, personal stories of skin cancer survivors, a section about skin cancer and skin of color, and the *Skin Cancer Foundation Journal*.

For Further Research

Books

Sarah L. Chamlin, *Living with Skin Conditions (Teen's Guides)*. New York: Facts On File, 2010.

Carrie Fredericks, *Skin Cancer*. Farmington Hills, MI: Gale Cengage, 2010.

Bonnie Juettner, *Acne*. Farmington Hills, MI: Gale Cengage, 2010.

Douglas B. Light, *Cells, Tissues, and Skin*. New York: Chelsea House, 2009.

Rebecca Penzer and Steven Ersser, *Principles of Skin Care*. West Sussex, England: Wiley, 2010.

Melanie Vasseur, *Under My Skin*. Campbell, CA: FastPencil, 2010.

Kim Wohlenhaus, *Skin Health Information for Teens*. Detroit, MI: Omnigraphics, 2009.

Periodicals

Debra D. Bass, "Fight Acne by Creating a Diversion," *Seattle Times*, July 3, 2011.

Jane E. Brody, "For Many Millions, Psoriasis Means Misery," *New York Times*, July 4, 2011.

Eleni N. Gage, "True or False: Most Sun Damage to Skin Is by Age 18," *Real Simple*, May 2010.

Laura Greenback, "Does Drinking Milk Cure Acne?," *Girls' Life*, April/May 2011.

Alice Park, "Cornering Skin Cancer," *Time*, June 20, 2011.

Karyn Repinski, "Finally! Sunscreens You'll Love to Wear!," *Prevention*, June 2009.

Alan Roberts, "Acne Attack: Every Teen Gets Pimples. Here's Why, and What to Do About It," *Scholastic Choices*, September 2009.

Dale Rodebaugh, "Man Recovering from Flesh-Eating Bacteria," *Durango (CO) Herald*, April 2, 2011.

Shannon Rossi, "It's Not Chicken Pox! Boy Has Rare Skin Disease," *Southgate (MI) News-Herald*, August 2, 2010.

Valerie Ulene, "Come on, It's Just Acne," *Chicago Tribune*, December 7, 2009.

Internet Sources

Acne.com, "Is It Really Acne?," 2011. www.acne.com/types-of-acne/is-it-really-acne.

Alain Gonzalez, "Working Out Causes Acne: TOP 5 Reasons!," Acne Teen, November 2009. www.acneteen.org/2009/11/working-out-causes-acne-top-5-reasons.html.

American Academy of Dermatology, "Skin of Color Population Faces Unique, but Treatable, Dermatologic Conditions," March 4, 2010. www.aad.org/stories-and-news/news-releases/skin-of-color-population-faces-unique-but-treatable-dermatologic-conditions.

Bruce Hensel, "Tanning Beds Lead to Increase in Teen Skin Cancer: Study," NBC San Diego, May 3, 2011. www.nbcsandiego.com/news/health/Tanning-Beds-Lead-to-Increase-in-Teen-Skin-Cancer-121190844.html.

MedicineNet, "Focus on Skin," Skin Health Center. www.medicinenet.com/skin/focus.htm.

Lynne Peeples, "Bad Acne Linked to Suicidal Thinking in Teens," CNN Health, September 16, 2010. www.cnn.com/2010/HEALTH/09/16/health.acne.suicidal.thinking/index.html.

US Environmental Protection Agency, *Health Effects of Overexposure to the Sun*, June 2010. www.epa.gov/sunwise/doc/healtheffects.pdf.

US Food and Drug Administration, "Facing Facts About Acne," *Consumer Health Information*, January 2010. www.fda.gov/downloads/ForConsumers/ConsumerUpdates/UCM197220.pdf.

———, "Indoor Tanning: The Risks of Ultraviolet Rays, *Consumer Health Information*, May 2010. www.fda.gov/downloads/ForConsumers/ConsumerUpdates/UCM190664.pdf.

Source Notes

Overview

1. Lucy Speed, "My Battle with Acne," interview by Kay Goddard, *Express*, August 10, 2010. www.express.co.uk.
2. Speed, "My Battle with Acne."
3. Speed, "My Battle with Acne."
4. Acne.com, "Skin Basics," 2011. www.acne.com.
5. Bernadine Healy, "Skin Deep," *U.S. News & World Report*, November 6, 2005. http://health.usnews.com.
6. National Institutes of Health, "Understanding Acne," *NIH News in Health*, January 2010. http://newsinhealth.nih.gov.
7. Quoted in Brian Donnolly, "Psoriasis: A Nuisance or a Deadly Disease?," FOX News, October 13, 2009. www.foxnews.com.
8. Quoted in National Rosacea Society, "The Great Impostor," July 12, 2011. www.rosacea.org.
9. Princeton University Health Services, "Skin Care," October 27, 2010. www.princeton.edu.
10. American Skin Association, "Melanoma," 2011. www.americanskin.org.
11. Seton Healthcare, "Acne: Cause," February 3, 2011. www.seton.net.
12. American Academy of Dermatology/AcneNet, "Adult Acne: A Fact of Life for Many Women," 2011. www.skincarephysicians.com.
13. Manny Alvarez, "Acne: The Scourge of the Teen Years," FOX News, January 9, 2007. www.foxnews.com.
14. James G.H. Dinulos, "Scabies," *Merck Manual Home Health Handbook*, September 2008. www.merckmanuals.com.
15. Skin Cancer Foundation, "UV Information: Understanding UVA and UVB," 2011. www.skincancer.org.
16. Robert J. MacNeal, "Diagnosis of Skin Disorders," *Merck Maual Home Health Handbook*, October 2006. www.merckmanuals.com.
17. Mayo Clinic, "Melanoma: Tests and Diagnosis," June 2, 2010. www.mayoclinic.com.
18. Alvarez, "Acne."
19. Quoted in *DermatologistsBlog*, "Updated Skin Care for Acne and Rosacea," February 4, 2011. http://dermatologistsblog.com.
20. American Academy of Dermatology, "Be Sun Smart," 2011. www.aad.org.

What Are Acne and Skin Disorders?

21. Seppo Puusa, "My Story," Clear for Life, March 2010. www.clear-for-life.com.
22. Puusa, "My Story."
23. Puusa, "My Story."
24. Alvarez, "Acne."
25. American Academy of Dermatology, "Early Acne Often Predicts Severe Acne," 2011. www.skincarephysicians.com.
26. John Grohol, "Acne Ups Teen Suicide Risk," PsychCentral, September 19, 2010. http://psychcentral.com.
27. Quoted in Grace Gold, "CariDee English Reveals Pictures of Her Painful Battle with Psoriasis: '70% of My Body Was Covered,'" Stylelist, June 4, 2010. www.stylelist.com.
28. Quoted in Gold, "CariDee English Reveals Pictures of Her Painful Battle with Psoriasis."
29. Quoted in Gold, "CariDee English Reveals Pictures of Her Painful Battle with Psoriasis."
30. Quoted in Gold, "CariDee English

Reveals Pictures of Her Painful Battle with Psoriasis."

31. Princeton University Health Services, "Skin Care."

32. Quoted in Drew Halfnight, "Giant Weed That Burns and Blinds Spreads Across Canada," *National Post*, July 13, 2010. http://news.nationalpost.com.

33. Princeton University Health Services, "Skin Care."

34. National Institutes of Health, "Basal Cell Carcinoma," February 5, 2008. www.ncbi.nlm.nih.gov.

35. National Institutes of Health, "Squamous Cell Skin Cancer," August 12, 2009. www.nlm.nih.gov.

36. Quoted in Zach Thaxton, "D-20 School Psychologist, 33, Dies from Melanoma," KOAA, December 2, 2010. www.koaa.com.

What Causes Acne and Skin Disorders?

37. Quoted in Katherine Faulkner, "Young Mother Used Sunbeds Five Times a Week . . . Now She Is Facing Death from Cancer," *Daily Mail*, June 19, 2010. www.dailymail.co.uk.

38. Quoted in Faulkner, "Young Mother Used Sunbeds Five Times a Week . . . Now She Is Facing Death from Cancer."

39. US Food and Drug Administration (FDA), "Indoor Tanning: The Risks of Ultraviolet Rays," May 2010. www.fda.gov.

40. Quoted in Nick Hanson, "U of M Study Definitively Links Indoor Tanning to Melanoma," news release, University of Minnesota Academic Health Center, May 27, 2010. www.ahc.umn.edu.

41. Angela Palmer, "Is Acne Caused by Heredity?," About.com: Acne, May 13, 2009. http://acne.about.com.

42. American Academy of Family Physicians, "Psoriasis," July 2010. http://familydoctor.org.

43. American Academy of Dermatology, "Acne Myths," January 30, 2009. www.skincarephysicians.com.

44. S. Zahra Ghodsi, Helmut Orawa, and Christos C. Zouboulis, "Prevalence, Severity, and Severity Risk Factors of Acne in High School Pupils: A Community-Based Study," *Journal of Investigative Dermatology*, March 12, 2009. www.nature.com.

45. Princeton University Health Services, "Skin Care."

46. American Academy of Dermatology, "Genital Warts: Who Gets and Causes," 2011. www.aad.org.

47. Mayo Clinic, "Genital Herpes," May 21, 2011. www.mayoclinic.com.

How Are Acne and Skin Disorders Treated?

48. Michael Khalili, "Vitiligo Has Me," *Michael Khalili* (blog), August 22, 2010. www.michaelapproved.com.

49. Khalili, "Vitiligo Has Me."

50. Khalili, "Vitiligo Has Me."

51. Quoted in *ScienceDaily*, "New Treatments and Good Skin Care Helping Patients Control Acne and Rosacea," March 8, 2010. www.sciencedaily.com.

52. Kayte Cook Watts, comment on Stephanie Wright, "Acne Files: Bad Breakout Stories Giveaway with Murad," *Beauty Blog*, DermStore, January 13, 2010. http://blog.dermstore.com.

53. WebMD, "Dermabrasion, Microdermabrasion, and Your Skin," February 25, 2011. www.webmd.com/healthy-beauty/dermabrasion-microdermabrasion.

54. Quoted in *ScienceDaily*, "New Treatments and Good Skin Care Helping Patients Control Acne and Rosacea."

55. Quoted in *ScienceDaily*, "New Treatments and Good Skin Care Helping

Patients Control Acne and Rosacea."

56. American Academy of Dermatology, "Skin Cancer: Diagnosis, Treatment, and Outcome," 2011. www.aad.org.

57. Melissa DeLuca Nowicki, "An Esthetician's Battle with Skin Cancer," Facebook, January 2011. www.facebook.com.

58. Mayo Clinic, "Plantar Warts: Treatment and Drugs," May 3, 2011. www.mayoclinic.com.

59. Quoted in Amy Harmon, "A Roller Coaster Chase for a Cure," *New York Times*, February 21, 2010. www.nytimes.com.

60. Quoted in Harmon, "A Roller Coaster Chase for a Cure."

Can Acne and Skin Disorders Be Prevented?

61. Jeanette M. Kamell et al. "Medical Students Educate Teens About Skin Cancer: What Have We Learned?," *Journal of Cancer Education*, April 27, 2010. www.ncbi.nlm.nih.gov.

62. Quoted in Kamell et al. "Medical Students Educate Teens About Skin Cancer."

63. Kamell, Rietkerk, Lam, Phillips, Wu, McCullough, Linden, and Osann, "Medical Students Educate Teens About Skin Cancer."

64. Mayo Clinic, "Skin Cancer: Prevention," August 18, 2010. www.mayoclinic.com.

65. Nowicki, "An Esthetician's Battle with Skin Cancer."

66. Nowicki, "An Esthetician's Battle with Skin Cancer."

67. Skin Cancer Foundation, "UV Information."

68. Mayo Clinic, "Dermatitis: Prevention," December 8, 2009. www.mayoclinic.com.

69. Mayo Clinic, "Dermatitis."

70. Mayo Clinic, "Acne: Prevention," November 3, 2009. www.mayoclinic.com.

71. American Academy of Dermatology, "Treating Acne in Skin of Color," 2011. www.skincarephysicians.com.

List of Illustrations

Index

Note: Boldface page numbers indicate illustrations.

About the Author

Peggy J. Parks holds a bachelor of science degree from Aquinas College in Grand Rapids, Michigan, where she graduated magna cum laude. An author who has written over 100 educational books for children and young adults, Parks lives in Muskegon, Michigan, a town that she says inspires her writing because of its location on the shores of Lake Michigan.